AF566942

PROGRESS IN CLINICAL AND BIOLOGICAL RESEARCH

RECENT TITLES

Vol 311: **Molecular and Cytogenetic Studies of Non-Disjunction,** Terry J. Hassold, Charles J. Epstein, *Editors*

Vol 312: **The Ocular Effects of Prostaglandins and Other Eicosanoids,** Laszlo Z. Bito, Johan Stjernschantz, *Editors*

Vol 313: **Malaria and the Red Cell: 2,** John W. Eaton, Steven R. Meshnick, George J. Brewer, *Editors*

Vol 314: **Inherited and Environmentally Induced Retinal Degenerations,** Matthew M. LaVail, Robert E. Anderson, Joe G. Hollyfield, *Editors*

Vol 315: **Muscle Energetics,** Richard J. Paul, Gijs Elzinga, Kazuhiro Yamada, *Editors*

Vol 316: **Hemoglobin Switching,** George Stamatoyannopoulos, Arthur W. Nienhuis, *Editors*. Published in two volumes: Part A: *Transcriptional Regulation*. Part B: *Cellular and Molecular Mechanisms*.

Vol 317: **Alzheimer's Disease and Related Disorders,** Khalid Iqbal, Henryk M. Wisniewski, Bengt Winblad, *Editors*

Vol 318: **Mechanisms of Chromosome Distribution and Aneuploidy,** Michael A. Resnick, Baldev K. Vig, *Editors*

Vol 319: **The Red Cell: Seventh Ann Arbor Conference,** George J. Brewer, *Editor*

Vol 320: **Menopause: Evaluation, Treatment, and Health Concerns,** Charles B. Hammond, Florence P. Haseltine, Isaac Schiff, *Editors*

Vol 321: **Fatty Acid Oxidation: Clinical, Biochemical, and Molecular Aspects,** Kay Tanaka, Paul M. Coates, *Editors*

Vol 322: **Molecular Endocrinology and Steroid Hormone Action,** Gordon H. Sato, James L. Stevens, *Editors*

Vol 323: **Current Concepts in Endometriosis,** Dev R. Chadha, Veasy C. Buttram, Jr., *Editors*

Vol 324: **Recent Advances in Hemophilia Care,** Carol K. Kasper, *Editor*

Vol 325: **Alcohol, Immunomodulation, and AIDS,** Daniela Seminara, Ronald Ross Watson, Albert Pawlowski, *Editors*

Vol 326: **Nutrition and Aging,** Derek M. Prinsley, Harold H. Sandstead, *Editors*

Vol 327: **Frontiers in Smooth Muscle Research,** Nicholas Sperelakis, Jackie D. Wood, *Editors*

Vol 328: **The International Narcotics Research Conference (INRC) '89,** Rémi Quirion, Khem Jhamandas, Christina Gianoulakis, *Editors*

Vol 329: **Multipoint Mapping and Linkage Based Upon Affected Pedigree Members: Genetic Analysis Workshop 6,** Robert C. Elston, M. Anne Spence, Susan E. Hodge, Jean W. MacCluer, *Editors*

Vol 330: **Verocytotoxin-Producing *Escherichia coli* Infections,** Martin Petric, Charles R. Smith, Clifford A. Lingwood, James L. Brunton, Mohamed A. Karmali, *Editors*

Vol 331: **Mouse Liver Carcinogenesis: Mechanisms and Species Comparisons,** Donald E. Stevenson, R. Michael McClain, James A. Popp, Thomas J. Slaga, Jerrold M. Ward, Henry C. Pitot, *Editors*

Vol 332: **Molecular and Cellular Regulation of Calcium and Phosphate Metabolism,** Meinrad Peterlik, Felix Bronner, *Editors*

Vol 333: **Bone Marrow Purging and Processing,** Samuel Gross, Adrian P. Gee, Diana A. Worthington-White, *Editors*

Vol 334: **Potassium Channels: Basic Function and Therapeutic Aspects,** Thomas J. Colatsky, *Editor*

Vol 335: **Evolution of Subterranean Mammals at the Organismal and Molecular Levels,** Eviatar Nevo, Osvaldo A. Reig, *Editors*

Vol 336: **Dynamic Interactions of Myelin Proteins,** George A. Hashim, Mario Moscarello, *Editors*

Vol 337: **Apheresis,** Gail Rock, *Editor*

Vol 338: **Hematopoietic Growth Factors in Transfusion Medicine,** Jerry Spivak, William Drohan, Douglas Dooley, *Editors*

Vol 339: **Advances in Cancer Control: Screening and Prevention Research,** Paul F. Engstrom, Barbara Rimer, Lee E. Mortenson, *Editors*

Vol 340: **Mutation and the Environment,** Mortimer L. Mendelsohn, Richard J. Albertini, *Editors*. Published in five volumes: Part A: *Basic Mechanisms*. Part B: *Metabolism, Testing Methods, and Chromosomes*. Part C: *Somatic and Heritable Mutation, Adduction, and Epidemiology*. Part D: *Carcinogenesis*. Part E: *Environmental Genotoxicity, Risk, and Modulation*.

Vol 341: **Chronobiology: Its Role in Clinical Medicine, General Biology, and Agriculture,** Dora K. Hayes, John E. Pauly, Russel J. Reiter, *Editors*. Published in two volumes.

Vol 342: **Progress in Comparative Endocrinology,** August Epple, Colin G. Scanes, Milton H. Stetson, *Editors*

Vol 343: **Horizons in Membrane Biotechnology,** Claude Nicolau, Dennis Chapman, *Editors*

Vol 344: **Isozymes: Structure, Function, and Use in Biology and Medicine,** Zen-Iichi Ogita, Clement L. Markert, *Editors*

Vol 345: **Sleep and Respiration,** Faiq G. Issa, Paul M. Suratt, John E. Remmers, *Editors*

Vol 346: **Recent Progress in Research on Nutrition and Cancer,** Curtis J. Mettlin, Kunio Aoki, *Editors*

Vol 347: **Mutagens and Carcinogens in the Diet,** Michael W. Pariza, Hans-Ulrich Aeschbacher, James S. Felton, Shigeaki Sato, *Editors*

Vol 348: **EORTC Genitourinary Group Monograph 9: Basic Research and Treatment of Renal Cell Carcinoma Metastasis,** C.G. Bollack, D. Jacqmin, *Editors*

Vol 349: **Cytokines and Lipocortins in Inflammation and Differentiation,** Marialuisa Melli, Luca Parente, *Editors*

Vol 350: **Uro-Oncology: Current Status and Future Trends,** H.G.W. Frohmüller, Manfred Wirth, *Editors*

Vol 351: **Taurine: Functional Neurochemistry, Physiology, and Cardiology,** Herminia Pasantes-Morales, David L. Martin, William Shain, Rafael Martìn del Rio, *Editors*

Vol 352: **The Biology of Hematopoiesis,** Nicholas Dainiak, Eugene P. Cronkite, Ronald McCaffrey, Richard K. Shadduck, *Editors*

Vol 353: **Neoadjuvant Chemotherapy in Invasive Bladder Cancer,** Ted A.W. Splinter, Howard I. Scher, *Editors*

Vol 354: **Effects of Therapy on Biology and Kinetics of the Residual Tumor,** Joseph Ragaz, Linda Simpson-Herren, Marc Lippman, Bernard Fisher, *Editors*. Published in two volumes: Part A: *Pre-Clinical Aspects*. Part B: *Clinical Aspects*.

Vol 355: **Radiolabelled Cellular Blood Elements,** Helmut Sinzinger, Mathew L. Thakur, *Editors*

Vol 356: **Molecular Biology and Differentiation of Megakaryocytes,** Janine Breton-Gorius, Jack Levin, Alan T. Nurden, Neil Williams, *Editors*

Vol 357: **EORTC Genitourinary Group Monograph 7: Prostate Cancer and Testicular Cancer,** W.G. Jones, Donald W.W. Newling, *Editors*

Vol 358: **Treatment of Post Surgical Adhesions,** Gere S. diZerega, L. Russell Malinak, Michael P. Diamond, Cary B. Linsky, *Editors*

Vol 359: **EORTC Genitourinary Group Monograph 8: Treatment of Prostatic Cancer—Facts and Controversies,** Fritz H. Schröder, *Editor*

Please contact publisher for information about previous titles in this series.

TREATMENT OF POST SURGICAL ADHESIONS

TREATMENT OF POST SURGICAL ADHESIONS

Proceedings of the First International Symposium for the Treatment of Post Surgical Adhesions, Held in Phoenix, Arizona, September 15–17, 1989

Editors

Gere S. diZerega
Department of Obstetrics and Gynecology
University of Southern California School of Medicine
Los Angeles, California

L. Russell Malinak
Department of Obstetrics and Gynecology
Baylor College of Medicine
Houston, Texas

Michael P. Diamond
Department of Obstetrics and Gynecology
Yale University School of Medicine
New Haven, Connecticut

Cary B. Linsky
Department of Clinical Research
Johnson & Johnson Medical, Inc.
New Brunswick, New Jersey

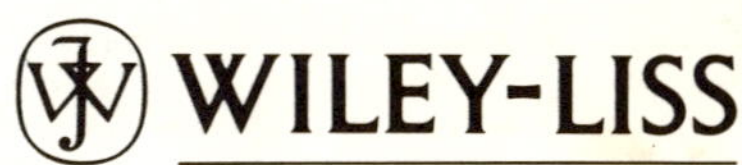

A JOHN WILEY & SONS, INC., PUBLICATION
NEW YORK • CHICHESTER • BRISBANE • TORONTO • SINGAPORE

Address all Inquiries to the Publisher
Wiley-Liss, Inc., 41 East 11th Street, New York, NY 10003

Printed in United States of America

The publication of this volume was facilitated by the authors and editors who submitted the text in a form suitable for direct reproduction without subsequent editing or proofreading by the publisher.

Library of Congress Cataloging-in-Publication Data

International Symposium for the Treatment of Post Surgical Adhesions (1st : 1989 : Phoenix, Ariz.)
Treatment of post surgical adhesions : proceedings of the First International Symposium for the Treatment of Post Surgical Adhesions, held in Phoenix, Arizona, September 15-17, 1989 / editors, Gere S. diZerega ... [et al.].
p. cm. -- (Progress in clinical and biological research ; v. 358)
Includes bibliographical references.
Includes index.
ISBN 0-471-56841-4
1. Adhesions--Prevention--Congresses. 2. Surgery--Complications and sequelae--Congresses. I. DiZerega, Gere S. II. Title. III. Series.
[DNLM: 1. Adhesions--therapy--congresses. 2. Postoperative Complications--congresses. W1 PR668E v. 358 / WI 900 I595t 1989]
RD647.A3I57 1989
617'.01--dc20
DNLM/DLC
for Library of Congress 90-12408
CIP

Contents

Contributors

Stephen P. Boyers, Division of Reproductive Biology and Medicine, Department of Obstetrics and Gynecology, University of California, Davis, CA 95616 **[93]**

Veasy C. Buttram, Jr., Department of Obstetrics and Gynecology, Baylor College of Medicine, Houston, TX 77030 **[113]**

Tim Cunningham, Johnson & Johnson Medical, Inc., New Brunswick, NJ 08903 **[131]**

Alan H. DeCherney, Department of Obstetrics and Gynecology, Division of Reproductive Endocrinology, Yale University School of Medicine, New Haven, CT 06510 **[145]**

Michael P. Diamond, Department of Obstetrics and Gynecology, Division of Reproductive Endocrinology, Yale University School of Medicine, New Haven, CT 06510 **[xi,23,131]**

Gere S. diZerega, Department of Obstetrics and Gynecology, University of Southern California School of Medicine, Livingston Reproductive Biology Laboratory, Los Angeles, CA 90033 **[xi,1]**

Randall C. Dunn, Department of Obstetrics and Gynecology, Baylor College of Medicine, Houston, TX 77030 **[113]**

Thomas E. Elkins, Department of Obstetrics and Gynecology, University of Michigan Medical Center, Ann Arbor, MI 48109 **[103]**

Robert W. Gracy, Department of Biochemistry, Tissue Repair Unit, University of North Texas, Texas College of Osteopathic Medicine, Fort Worth, TX 76107 **[131]**

Avner Hershlag, Department of Obstetrics and Gynecology, Division of Reproductive Endocrinology, Yale University School of Medicine, New Haven, CT 06510 **[23]**

Jaroslav F. Hulka, Department of Obstetrics and Gynecology, University of North Carolina, Chapel Hill, NC 27514 **[13]**

David Jansen, Woody Mountain Facility, Medical Products, W.L. Gore and Associates, Inc., Flagstaff, AZ 86002 **[93]**

The numbers in brackets are the opening page numbers of the contributors' articles.

Robert P.S. Jansen, Department of Fertility Services, Royal Prince Alfred Hospital, Sydney 2050, Australia [177]

Lola Kamp, Johnson & Johnson Patient Care, New Brunswick, NJ 08903 [131]

William R. Keye, Jr., Department of Obstetrics and Gynecology, University of Utah Health Sciences Center, Salt Lake City, UT 84132 [67]

Bertil Larsson, Department of Obstetrics and Gynecology, Karolinska Institutet, Huddinge University Hospital, S-14186 Huddinge, Sweden [165]

Carl J. Levinson, Department of Obstetrics, Gynecology, and Reproductive Sciences, University of California San Francisco and Children's Hospital San Francisco, San Francisco, CA 94118 [45]

Cary B. Linsky, Department of Clinical Research, Johnson & Johnson Medical, Inc., New Brunswick, NJ 08903 [xi,131]

Anthony A. Luciano, Departments of Obstetrics and Gynecology and Reproductive Endocrinology, University of Connecticut School of Medicine, Farmington, CT 06032 [35]

L. Russell Malinak, Department of Obstetrics and Gynecology, Baylor College of Medicine, Houston, TX 77030 [xi,193]

Robert F. McConnell, Consultant Pathologist, Flemington, NJ 76107 [131]

William R. Meyer, Department of Obstetrics and Gynecology, Division of Reproductive Endocrinology, Yale University School of Medicine, New Haven, CT 06510 [145]

Kathleen E. Rodgers, Department of Obstetrics and Gynecology, University of Southern California School of Medicine, Los Angeles, CA 90033 [119]

Sanford M. Rosenberg, Richmond Center for Fertility and Endocrinology, Ltd., Richmond, VA 23229 [157]

Richard M. Soderstrom, Department of Obstetrics and Gynecology, University of Washington Medical School, Seattle, WA 98122 [59]

J. Baptist Trimbos, Department of Gynecology and Reproduction, Leiden University Medical Centre, Leiden 2333 AA, The Netherlands [77]

Trudy C.M. Trimbos-Kemper, Department of Gynecology and Reproduction, Leiden University Medical Centre, Leiden 2333 AA, The Netherlands [77]

Togas Tulandi, Department of Obstetrics and Gynecology, McGill University, Montreal, Quebec H3A 1A1, Canada [85]

Eylard V. van Hall, Department of Gynecology and Reproduction, Leiden University Medical Centre, Leiden 2333 AA, The Netherlands [77]

Preface

As a result of the expanding research in post surgical peritoneal repair and prevention of adhesion formation that occurred in the 1980s, a group of clinicians, academicians, and medical industry representatives formed an ad hoc committee to facilitate communication of this multidisciplinary research. As a consequence, on September 15–17, 1989, the First International Symposium for the Treatment of Post Surgical Adhesions was convened in Phoenix, Arizona. Speakers were invited to summarize recent data based on their contemporary contributions to the field. This monograph brings together their manuscripts in an attempt to capture state-of-the-art research under one cover.

An overview of the general process of post surgical repair of the peritoneum is compared to the better known process of skin repair. The difficulties encountered in classifying adhesions for the purpose of study and quantitative analysis are identified and an array of potentially useful systems critiqued.

Differences in the response to treatment of adhesions that form de novo, in contrast to those that reform after lysis, are highlighted, and therapeutic consequences are considered. A full array of data and conclusions are provided to address the options of surgical techniques, including the role of laparoscopic surgery in comparison to traditional laparotomy approaches and the use of lasers in intraperitoneal surgery. The controversy of second-look laparoscopy is reviewed from the viewpoint of the patient's clinical benefit.

Over the last decade a variety of adjuvants to surgical therapy for adhesion prevention were introduced to pelvic surgeons or underwent animal studies with varying degree of success. These include dextran, surgical barriers, corticosteroids, heparin, nonsteroidal anti-inflammatory drugs, fibrinolytics, hydrogels, and procoagulants. The above-mentioned surgical procedures, adjuvants, and strategies were placed into perspective with recent advances in alternative reproductive technologies to provide an overview of the contributions and limitations that these new procedures and medicaments continue to make in the surgical arena. The clinical investigators and scientists who provided important data for each of these modalities present here an up-to-date summary of the role that each of these technologies may play in reproductive surgery.

Gere S. diZerega, M.D.
L. Russell Malinak, M.D.
Michael P. Diamond, M.D.
Cary B. Linsky, Ph.D.

Treatment of Post Surgical Adhesions, pages 1–11

THE PERITONEUM AND ITS RESPONSE TO SURGICAL INJURY

Gere S. diZerega, M.D.
Department Obstetric and Gynecology, University of Southern California School of Medicine
Livingston Reproductive Biology Laboratory
1321 North Mission Road
Los Angeles, California 90033

The peritoneum is a serous membrane of mesodermal origin which lines the walls of the abdomen (parietal peritoneum) and is reflected over the viscera (visceral peritoneum). The peritoneum forms a closed sac in the male and an open sac in the female since the ends of the fallopian tubes and ovaries are not covered by peritoneum. It consists of mesothelial cells in a continuous layer which rest upon loose mesenchymal tissue, a basal lamina, and basement membrane composed of a collagen lattice. The connective tissue is arranged into bundles which interlace in a plane parallel to the surface. There are numerous elastic fibers, especially in the deeper layer of the parietal peritoneum, and comparatively few connective tissue cells. The loose connective tissue of the peritoneum may contain collagen and elastin fibers, fibroblasts, macrophages, lymphocytes, plasma cells, eosinophils, mast cells, fat cells and blood vessels.

Pfeiffer et al., (1987) described the ultrastructure of the visceral peritoneum covering the stomach, small intestine and colon of the immature pig as a single layer of loosely attached squamous epithelial cells which contain microvilli and are loosely attached to the underlying connective tissue. Adjacent mesothelial cells are joined either by desmosomes or are loosely connected at their peripheral edges. The apical surface of the mesothelial cells contain an abundance of long microvilli so that the entire surface area of the peritoneum is generally equal to that of the skin. A role for mesothelial microvilli in transport function is suggested by the absorptive and exudative ability of the mesothelium (Andrews and Porter, 1973).

The peritoneum contains a basement membrane which consists of a delicate fibrillar plexus and a plexus of reticulum fibers. The orientation of the reticulum and fibroblasts is longitudinal to the plan of expansion appropriate for the anatomical site. Connection of the peritoneum to the basement membrane involves an underlying network of elastin, collagen and glycosaminoglycans. The deep latticed collagenous layer of the basement membranes is separated from the superficial collagen by a network of elastin. Above this are "layers" of vascular tissue, deep collagen and mucopolysaccarides, elastin, connective or mesenchymal tissue, superficial collagen, and mesothelial cells.

The peritoneum is supplied with blood vessels and lymphatics which give rise to a rich capillary network. In the adult blood and lymphatic vessels of the peritoneum are found in the deep latticed collagenous layer. The deepest vessels of the peritoneum are parallel with the musculature underlying the peritoneum. More superficial vessels, penetrating to the thickness of the deep collagenous layer, are parallel with the spiral arterioles which precludes over extension of the vessels which may occur during peritoneal stretching. Blood vessels of the mesentary or intestinal peritoneum contain adventitial sheaths: elastin for the arteries; collagen for the veins.

Parietal peritoneum is innervated by branches of the spinal nerves which supply the abdominal wall. Peritoneal involvement in visceral disease provides pain sensation through the lower intercostal nerves. Sensory supply to the parietal peritoneum covering the diaphragm involves both the phrenic nerves as well as the intercostals. Diaphragmatic pain may be perceived either at the base of the neck or shoulder (from C_3, C_4, and C_5 via the phrenic nerves) or in the abdominal wall. Pain fibers have not been clearly shown for visceral peritoneum. Visceral pain is perceived via the viscus itself or from stretch or spasm of the visceral smooth muscles.

The peritoneum serves to minimize friction facilitating free movement between abdominal viscera, resist localized infection, and store fat especially in the greater omentum.

Peritoneal Repair

It was shown in 1919 that peritoneal healing differs from that of skin (Hertzler, 1949). When a defect is made in the parietal peritoneum "the entire surface becomes endothelialized simultaneously and not gradually from the borders as in epidermidalization of skin wounds". Peritoneal defects 2 x 2 cm and 0.5 x 0.5 cm were both entirely covered by a continuous sheet of mesothelium 3 days after wounding. The granulation and contraction that occurs around the edges of skin wounds does not occur during peritoneal healing.

Ellis et al. (1975) identified an early and late phase of cellular morphology in peritoneal repair. Initially, an inflammatory exudate develops that includes polymorphonuclear leukocytes (PMNs), histocytes, and monocytes in a fibrin exudate. Within 48-72 hours after surgically induced peritoneal injury, these cells are replaced by fibroblasts, which then secrete collagen beneath the peritoneal surface.

Raftery (1973b) evaluated postsurgical healing of both parietal and visceral peritoneum in rats after excision as well as abrasion of peritoneum. During the first 2 days wounds were grossly evident as they were uneven and hemorrhagic. By 5 days they were smooth and glistening. Wounds of the parietal peritoneum over the liver capsule remained through day 10 as shiny, grayish-white, puckered areas. In contrast, wounds of the parietal peritoneum were difficult to identify after 7 days. After 5 days it was difficult to see the wounds of the cecum where peritoneum was previously stripped off the surface.

Some discrepancy exists between various studies on the time taken for regeneration of the mesothelial layer. Ellis et al. (1965) and Hubbard et al. (1967) reported that re-epithelialization of parietal peritoneum occurs in 5-6 days. Glucksman (1966) showed that visceral mesothelium covering the terminal ileum re-epithelializes in 5 days, while Eskeland (1966a) found that regeneration of the mesothelium of parietal peritoneum is not complete until 8 days. Raftery (1973b) confirmed the findings of Eskeland (1966a,b) in that parietal peritoneum of the rat is re-epithelialized by 8 days. While multiplication and migration of mesothelial cells from the margin of the wound may play a small part in the regenerative process it cannot play a major role, since new mesothelium develops in the center of a large wound at the same time as it develops in the center of a smaller one.

Raftery (1973a) studied the regeneration of parietal and visceral peritoneum using electron microscopic evaluation of healing peritoneal defects in the rat. Twelve hours after injury, numerous PMNs were seen entangled in fibrin strands (Figure 1). Very little cellular infiltrate was found in the depths of the wound compared to the wound surface. At 24-36 hrs after wounding the number of cells in the superficial part of the wound was greatly increased due to infiltration by macrophages. The macrophages were intertwined with filaments of fibrin projecting from the wound surface while the base of the wound remained relatively acellular. At 2 days most of the wound surface was covered with a single layer of macrophages supported by a fibrin scaffold. Two additional cell types were also seen on the wound surface: a cell which looked like a primitive mesenchymal cell found in small numbers at the wound base and mesothelial cells which formed islands within the peritoneal injury. The islets of mesothelial cells were interconnected by desmosomes and tight junctions. At 3 days the number of primitive mesenchymal cells on the wound surface increased although macrophages were still the most prevalent cell type present. The base of the wound contained scattered mesenchymal cells and some proliferating fibroblasts. The cells on the wound surface at 3 days were similar in appearance to the primitive mesenchymal cells located in the deeper layers of the wound. At 4 days cells resembling primitive mesenchymal cells or proliferating fibroblasts on the wound surface came into contact with one another. In some areas re-epithelialization appeared complete at 5 days since a single layer of mesothelial cells was present on the wound surface interconnected by desmosomes and tight junctions. No basement membrane was seen beneath the mesothelial cells of parietal peritoneum or caecum at this stage, although one was often present beneath those covering the liver. Thus, peritoneal healing of parietal peritoneum was associated with basement

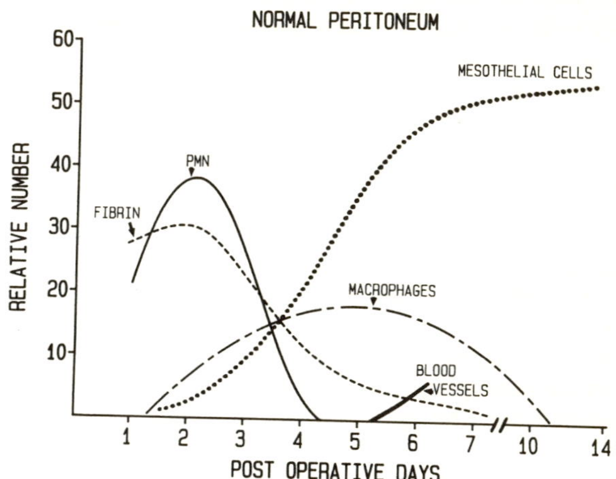

Figure 1

Change in the relative number of cellular elements and fibrinolysis (fibrin) at the site of peritoneal injury in mature rats during the course of re-epithelialization. (Summarized from Bridges and Whitting, 1964; Ellis et al., 1965; Eskeland and Kjærheim, 1966a; Johnson and Whitting, 1962; Raftery 1973a,b).

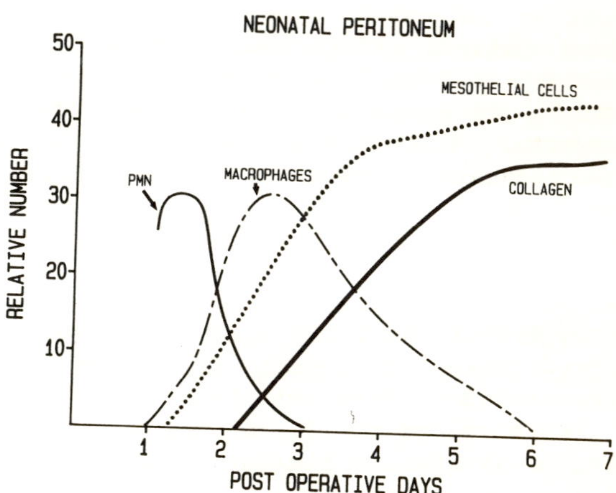

Figure 2

Change in the relative number of cellular elements and collagen production at the site of peritoneal injury in mature rats during the course of re-epithelialization (Summarized from Ellis et al., 1965; Raftery 1973c).

membrane formation in contrast to visceral peritoneum which although similar in appearance on the surface, frequently did not involve healing of the basement membrane. In other areas healing was far less advanced demonstrating some variability in the rate of cellular response.

Eskeland and Kjærheim (1966a) described the cellular sequence of repair in the parietal peritoneum of rats after either burn or stripping of the peritoneum off the body wall. Both small and large wounds contained a continuous layer of mesothelial cells 8 days after injury. Wounds which measured 36 mm in diameter were completely covered with new mesothelium at day 8. The intact peritoneum adjacent to the wound (1-3 mm) formed the second day after injury. Outside of this area, the number of dividing cells rapidly decreased while away from the wound, few or no cells were observed in mitosis. A high mitotic activity was also found in the surface cells within the wound. Cells in division were occasionally seen at day 3, and they reached maximum number at day 4 and day 6. At day 8, a considerable number of cells were seen in division within the limits of the wound, while mitotic activity in the mesothelium outside the wound had almost ceased.

Visceral Peritoneum

Visceral peritoneum appears to differ little in its healing properties from the parietal peritoneum. Raftery (1973a) reported that the liver acquired a new mesothelial covering one day earlier than either caecum or parietal peritoneum. A discontinuous basement membrane was seen beneath the mesothelial cell layer of visceral peritoneum at 5 days. In contrast, basement membrane was not seen beneath the mesothelial cells of the parietal peritoneum or caecum until 7 days. Raftery hypothesized that the liver (viscera) provides a firmer substrate for development of new mesothelium than either the parietes or caecum, both of which are more subject to distension.

Drying Injury

Prolonged drying of the peritoneum was shown by Ryan et al. (1971) to induce significant injury. Immediately after drying, intact mesothelial cells were found to be absent in a rat cecal preparation. Four hours later, no mesothelial cells were seen; most of the surface showed only an irregular thin coating of fibrin without cells. In some areas aggregations of fibrin entrapped mononuclear cells, mast cells and eosinophils. The underlying muscle coat contained gross edema, cellular disintegration and partial occlusion of blood vessels by platelet masses.

Neonate

Intestinal obstruction due to adhesion formation was reported to occur more commonly after abdominal surgery in the infant or neonate in comparison to the adult (Devens, 1963; Replogle, Johnson, Gross, 1966). Ellis, Harrison and Hugh (1965) reported that peritoneal repair occurred more rapidly in the immature rat than in mature animals. Raftery (1973c) described the healing of visceral and parietal peritoneum in the immature rat at various times after standardized surgical injury (Figure 2). Although the wounds looked hemorrhagic and uneven 24 hours after injury, they were smooth and glistening at 3 days, and usually indistinguishable from the normal surrounding parietal peritoneum at 5 days. The cellular changes which accompanied these gross morphological changes were the same as those described for the adult rat except that mesothelial regeneration occurred more rapidly. By 2 days after injury, the acute inflammatory response had subsided leaving primarily macrophages and fibroblasts on the wound surface.

Active fibroblast proliferation occurred at the base of the wound. By 5 days the number of macrophages diminished leaving only fibroblasts. These fibroblasts came together to form the new mesothelium by 7 days compared with 8 days in the adult. In the case of visceral peritoneum, mesothelial regeneration was complete by 5 days compared to 7 days in the adult rat. Again, there was no difference in the rate of healing between large and small peritoneal defects. Ellis et al. (1965) confirmed that re-epithelialization occurred faster in immature compared to mature rats. The defect in the parietal peritoneum acquired a smooth surface by 48 hr, and at 5 days the site of wounding was difficult to discern.

Mesothelial Cell Origin

Some investigators consider that metaplasia of fibroblasts within the loose connective tissue beneath the surface of the peritoneum leads to mesothelial regeneration (Robbins et al., 1949; Williams, 1955; Ellis et al., 1965; Hubbard et al., 1967). Others suggest that cells detach from the adjacent intact peritoneum and become implanted on the wound surface where they proliferate to form a continuous layer of mesothelium, (Johnson and Whitting, 1962; Bridges and Whitting, 1964). General agreement exists that peritoneal defects are covered by the immigration of mesothelial cells from the intact peritoneum bordering the wound. Mesothelial cells detach from adjacent peritoneum and implant on the wound surface as free grafts which then proliferate to form a new syncytium.

Origin of New Mesothelial Cells

Wide spread agreement exists that large defects heal as quickly as small defects so that repair does not occur by "granulation" of cells adjacent to the wound as happens in skin repair. The origin of new mesothelium is unclear because of difficulty in distinguishing between primitive mesenchymal cells and proliferating fibroblasts in the later stages of healing. It is possible that the former give rise to the latter, but definitive evidence for this is lacking. Possible origins of new mesothelium include:

(a) Transformation of underlying undifferentiated mesenchymal cells into new peritoneum (Robbins, Brunschwig & Foote, 1949; Williams, 1955; Hubbard et al., 1967; Ellis, 1963; Ellis, Harrison & Hugh, 1965; Bridges & Whitting, 1964).

(b) Transplantation of cells from peritoneal surfaces of adjacent viscera; Johnson & Whitting, 1962; Bridges & Whitting, 1964).

(c) Transformation of cells in the peritoneal fluid to mesothelial cells (Eskeland, 1966; Eskeland & Kjærheim, 1966a,b).

(d) Growth from cells at the periphery of the

defect (Johnson & Whitting, 1962; Bridges & Whitting, 1964; Ellis et al., 1965; Eskeland, 1966; Hubbard et al., 1967).

Ellis et al. (1965) reasoned that peritoneal reepithelialization results from the transformation of subperitoneal fibroblasts into an intact mesothelium. This is supported by the work of Robbins et al. (1949) and Williams (1955), who suggested that new peritoneum arose from the transformation of underlying connective tissue cells. Ellis' work was confirmed by Buckman et al. (1976), who reported that attempts to close over areas of peritoneal injury also prevented autolysis of early fibrinous attachments, and led to increased adhesion formation at the sites of reperitonealization. Since primitive mesencyhmal cells were present on both the surface of the wound and in its base during the early stages of healing, at least some of the new peritoneum appears to arise by metaplasia of subperitoneal fibroblasts (Raftery, 1973a,b).

References

Andrews PM, Porter KR (1973). The ultrastructural morphology and possible functional significance of mesothelial microvilli. Anat Res 177:408-426.

Bridges JB, Johnson FR, Whitting HW (1965). Peritoneal adhesion formation. Acta Anat (Basel) 61:203-212.

Bridges JB, Whitting HW (1964). Parietal peritoneal healing in the rat. J Path Bact 87:123-130.

Buckman RF, Woods M, Sargent L, Gervin AS (1976). A unifying pathogenetic mechanism in the aetiology of intraperitoneal adhesions. J Surg Res 20:1-5.

Buckman RF, Buckman PD, Hufnagel HV, Gervin AS (1976). A physiologic basis for the adhesion-free healing of deperitonealized surfaces. J Surg Res 21:67-76.

Devens K (1963). "Recurrent intestinal obstruction in the neonatal period." Archs Dis Childh 38:118-119.

Ellis H (1963). The aetiology of post-operative abdominal adhesions: an experimental study. Brit J Surg 50:10-16.

Ellis H, Harrison W, Hugh TB (1965). The healing of peritoneum under normal and pathological conditions. Brit J Surg 52:471-476.

Ellis H (1971). The cause and prevention of postoperative intraperitoneal adhesions. Surgery Gynec Obstet

133:497-511.

Eskeland G (1966). Growth of autologous peritoneal cells in intraperitoneal diffusion chambers in rats. I. A light microscopical study. Acta Pathol Microbiol Scandinav 68:481-500.

Eskeland G, Kjærheim Å (1966a). Regeneration of parietal peritoneum in rats. I. A light microscopical study. Acta Pathol Microbiol Scandinav 68:353-378.

Eskeland G, Kjærheim Å (1966b). Regeneration of parietal peritoneum in rats. II. An electron microscopical study. Acta Path Microbiol Scandinav 68:379-395.

Eskeland G, Kjærheim Å (1966c). Growth of autologogous peritoneal fluid cells in intraperitoneal diffusion chambers in rats. II. An electron microscopical study. Acta Pathol Microbiol Scandinav 68:501-516.

Glucksman DL, Warren WD (1966). The effect of topically applied corticosteroids in the prevention of peritoneal adhesions: an experimental approach with a review of the literature. Surgery 60:352-360.

Hertzler, AE (1919). "The Peritoneum." St. Louis: CV Mosby.

Hubbard TB, Khan MZ, Carag VR, Albites VE, Hricko GM (1967). The pathology of peritoneal repair: its relation to the formation of adhesions. Ann Surg 165:908-916.

Johnson FR, Whitting HW (1962). Repair of parietal peritoneum. Brit J Surg 49:653-660.

Pfeiffer CJ, Pfeiffer DC, Misra HP (1987). Enteric serosal surface in the piglet. A scanning and transmission electron microscopic study of the mesothelium. J Submicrosc Cytol 19:237-246.

Raftery AT (1973a). Regeneration of parietal and visceral peritoneum: an electron microscopical study. J Anat 115:375-392.

Raftery AT (1973b). Regeneration of parietal and visceral peritoneum. A light microscopical study. Br J Surg 60:293-299.

Raftery AT (1973c). Regeneration of parietal and visceral peritoneum in the immature animal: a light and electron microscopical study. Br J Surg 60:969-975.

Replogle RL, Johnson R, Gross RE (1966). Prevention of postoperative intestinal adhesions with combined promethazine and dexamethazone therapy: experimental and clinical studies. Ann Surg 163:580-588.

Robbins GF, Brunschwig A, Foote FW (1949). Deperitonealization: clinical and experimental observations. Ann.

Surg. 130:466-479, 1949.

Ryan GB, Grobety J, Majno G (1971). Postoperative peritoneal adhesions: a study of the mechanisms. Am J Pathol 64:117-148.

Williams DC (1955). The peritoneum. A plea for a change in attitude towards this membrane. Brit J Surg 42:401-405.

Treatment of Post Surgical Adhesions, pages 13–21

STAGING OF ADNEXAL ADHESIONS: A BRIEF HISTORY

Jaroslav F. Hulka M.D.

Professor of Obstetrics and Gynecology
University of North Carolina
Chapel Hill, NC 27514

In the mid 1970's , the emergence of microsurgery in the United States as a means of treating previously inoperable adnexal adhesions stirred interest in both the surgery itself and the evaluation of results. It soon became apparent that a system for classification of patients based on staging the initial disease found would be necessary to evaluate these new surgical techniques, This article will briefly review these efforts.

(In this discussion CLASSIFICATION applies to patients for purposes of scientific comparison: the nature of the disease, the extent of the disease, the operation performed, and the presence of other factors all influence to which category a patient belongs. STAGING applies to a system describing the extent of a disease.)

I. SURGICAL CLASSIFICATION: The Palmer System. In 1977 about 30 microsurgeons from throughout the world met to discuss classification during the Ninth World Congress of Fertility and Sterility. There was overwhelming consensus that an agreement should be reached on a classification system. Although no system was arrived at during the meeting, Dr. Raoul Palmer later circulated his system of classification ofsurgery among these participants. This was published by Siegler (1979) and is widely used as the standard classification of infertility surgery (see Table 1).

Table I: Classification of Surgical Techniques

I. Implantation
   A. Isthmus
   B. Ampulla

II. Anastomosis
   A. Intramural (interstitial)
      1. Isthmus
      2. Ampulla
   B. Ampulla
      1. Ampulla

III. Salpingostomy
   A. Terminal
   B. Midampulla (medial)
   C. Isthmus (included linear salpingoneostomy)

IV. Fimbrioplasty
   A. Deagglutination and/or dilatation
   B. Incision of peritoneal ring
   C. Incision of tubal wall

V. Lysis of adhesions (classified according to adnexa with mildest adhesions)
   A. Mild (less than 1 cm of tube or ovary involved in band or strings)
   B. Moderate (partially surrounding tube or ovary)
   C. Severe (encapsulating peritubal or periovarian adhesions)

VI. Combinations
   A. Different operations on right or left tubes
   B. Multiple operations on same tube (i.e., implantation and anastomosis)

Ad Hoc Committee of the Ninth World Congress of Fertility and Sterility, April 12-16, 1977, Miami Beach, FL.

Limitations: It is important to note that this does not describethe extent of disease found,nor does it describe the disease itself (eg: Endometriosis vs. iatrogenic adhesions vs. inflammatory adhesions). Nevertheless, this is an enormously useful classification of surgery performed.

II. DESCRIPTIVE CLASSIFICATION: The American Fertility Society (AFS) Systems. The AFS Endometriosis Committee has proposed a system for recording the findings at surgery of endometriosis where the extent and size of endometriomas are recorded together with the extent of ovarian and tubal involvement with adhesions. the nature of the adhesions (filmy or dense) is also evaluated. The most recently revised system has a score range of 1 to over 40.

This system is the basis for the AFS 1988 Ad Hoc Committee recommendation for a Classification of Adnexal Adhesions (Figure 1). This Committee adapted the description of adhesions used in the endometriosis classification , with two important additions:

1. Describing the left and right adnexa separately,
2. Estimates of prognosis by the surgeon based on the adnexum with the least ammount of pathology.

Limitations: The evaluation of this system to define categories as prognostic indicators awaits further prospective trials or retrospective analyses, but it does represent the current consensus of the AFS.

III. PROGNOSTIC CLASSIFICATION: In 1982 I published a system of staging adnexal adhesions based on a retrospective analysis of pregnancies after microsurgery. The extent of the adhesions was correlated with outcome as defined by subsequent term birth. During the analysis two factors emerged as correllating with pregnancy outcome: the extent of ovarian surface involvement, and the nature of the adhesions themselves. They were arbitrarily assigned two stages each:

I or II: less than half or more than half of the ovary surface involved,

A or B: filmy or dense adhesions.

Each adnexum was staged separately, and the adnexum with the least disease was used to classify the patient for comparison purposes.

FIGURE 1

THE AMERICAN FERTILITY SOCIETY CLASSIFICATION OF ADNEXAL ADHESIONS

Patient's Name ______________________ Date ________ Chart # ________

Age ______ G ______ P ______ Sp Ab ______ VTP ______ Ectopic ______ Infertile Yes ______ No ______

Other Significant History (i.e. surgery, infection, etc.) ______________________

____

HSG ________ Sonography ________ Photography ________ Laparoscopy ________ Laparotomy ________

	ADHESIONS	<1/3 Enclosure	1/3 - 2/3 Enclosure	>2/3 Enclosure
OVARY	R Filmy	1	2	4
	Dense	4	8	16
	L Filmy	1	2	4
	Dense	4	8	16
TUBE	R Filmy	1	2	4
	Dense	4*	8*	16
	L Filmy	1	2	4
	Dense	4*	8*	16

* If the fimbriated end of the fallopian tube is completely enclosed, change the point assignment to 16.

Prognostic Classification for Adnexal Adhesions

	LEFT		RIGHT
A. Minimal	________	0-5	________
B. Mild	________	6-10	________
C. Moderate	________	11-20	________
D. Severe	________	21-32	________

Treatment (Surgical Procedures): ______________________

____

____

____

____

Prognosis for Conception & Subsequent Viable Infant**

______ Excellent (> 75%)

______ Good (50-75%)

______ Fair (25%-50%)

______ Poor (< 25%)

** Physician's judgment based upon adnexa with least amount of pathology.

Recommended Followup Treatment: ______________________

____

____

Additional Findings: ______________________

____

____

____

____

____

DRAWING

L R

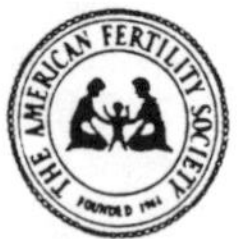

Property of
The American Fertility Society

For additional supply write to:
The American Fertility Society
2140 11th Avenue, South
Suite 200
Birmingham, Alabama 35205

More factors are involved in determining pregnancy outcome than just the extent of adhesions. The nature of the disease (endometriosis vs. PID) and extent of tubal damage (distal and/or proximal occlusion) and other fertility factors are also important. For these reasons the system included both tubal disease and adnexal adhesions (Figure 2).

Figure 2
Prognostic Staging of Adnexal Disease

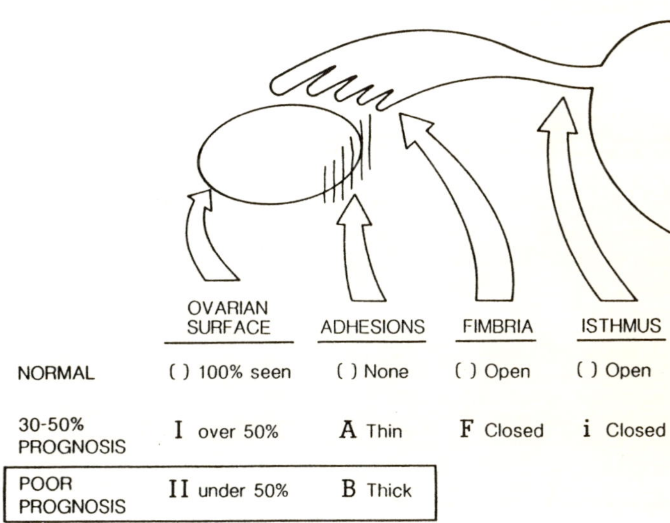

	OVARIAN SURFACE	ADHESIONS	FIMBRIA	ISTHMUS
NORMAL	( ) 100% seen	( ) None	( ) Open	( ) Open
30-50% PROGNOSIS	I over 50%	A Thin	F Closed	i Closed
POOR PROGNOSIS	II under 50%	B Thick		

After I arrived at this system by retrospective analysis I found that it was similar to a system suggested by Caspi (1979). He also found that both the extent of ovarian surface involvement (small versus large areas) and the nature of the adhesions (thin verses thick) were important. Table 2 presents his system. Table 3 presents pregnancies in these two series analyzed by these similar systems: pregnancy rates and deliveries decreased as these stages of adhesive disease increased .

I would now like to propose that a simple system for describing adhesive disease with only four stages would be adequate for current clinical prognostic needs as presented in table 4.

Table 2

CASPI SYSTEM
(Prognostic Value)

	Grade
Localized, fine, avascular, small areas	I
Extensive, " " large "	II
Localized, fibrous, vascular, small areas	III
Extensive, " " large "	IV

Caspi E, . . Fert Ster 31:296:1979

Table 3

STAGING SYSTEMS:
PROGNOSTIC VALUE

Caspi Series (n=42)		Hulka Series (n=47)	
Grade	Pregnancy %	Stage	Delivery%
I	71	I A	47
II	50	I B	44
III	28	II A	12
IV	20	II B	0

Table 4

SIMPLIFIED ADHESION CLASSIFICATION:

	Filmy	Dense
Less than 1/2 ovary enclosed	I	II
More than 1/2 ovary enclosed	III	IV

Prognosis (estimate)		
	I - 50-75%	Classify each adnexum separately
	II - 25-50%	
	III - 12-25%	
	IV - 0-12%	Prognosis based on best adnexum

Limitations: This system does not include the nature of the disease process (endometriosis versus PID) nor does it take into account tubal pathology or other fertility factors, conditions which require even more categories. For statistically meaningful comparisons, the number of patients in any category needs to be large, and practicality dictates that the number of categories should be kept to a minimum. For these reasons the number of stages in describing adhesions should be kept to a minimum.

IV. EXPERIMENTAL CLASSIFICATIONS: Systems for staging the extent of both human and animal adhesions have been devised to evaluate experimental techniques to reduce adhesion re-formation. These systems range from a simple "grade 0-3" system proposed by Siegler (1980) for experimentally induced adhesions in animals, to a clinical scoring of tubes and ovaries from 4 to 16 based on extent of organ involvement (diZerega 1983). A detailed experimental staging based on both the appearance of adhesions and their resistance to lysis was used by Boyers et al (1988).

Limitations: The degree of descriptive detail required for scientific evaluation of experiments in adhesion prevention runs counter to the long range need to keep categories to a minimum clinically.

Summary: Arriving at a system for staging adnexal disease is a scientific, clinical and political process which has already begun. Gynecologic oncologists started this process in 1967, and are still arriving at refinements and adjustments in the staging of cancer after 22 years. To rigorously evaluate new medical and surgical technologies in the treatment of adhesions it is important for infertility surgeons to continue the process of working towards a classification system, keeping in mind that it will take a long time.

References:

Adhesion Study Group (diZerega, GS),(1983). Reduction of postoperative pelvic adhesions with intraperitoneal 32% dextran 70: a prospective, randomized clinical trial. Fert Ster 40:612-619.

The American Fertility Society (Buttram Jr VC) (1988). The American Fertility Society Classification Of Anexal Adhesions, Distal Tubal Occlusion, Tubal Occlusion, Secondary To Tubal Ligation, Tubal Pregnancies, Mullerian Anomalies And Intrauterine Adhesions. Fert Ster 49:944-955.

Boyers SP, Diamond MP, DeCherney AH (1988). Reduction of postoperative pelvic adhesions in the rabbit with Gore-Tex* surgical membrane. Fert Ster 49:1066-1070.

Caspi E, Halperin Y, Bukovsky I (1979). The Importance Of Periadnexal Adhesions In Tubal Reconstructive Surgery For Infertility. Fert Ster 31:296-300.

Hulka, JF (1982) Adnexal adhesions: A prognostic staging and classification system based on a five-year survey of fertility surgery results at Chapel Hill, North Carolina. Am J Obstet Gynecol 144:141-148.

Siegler AM, Kontopoulos V, (1979). An Analysis Of Macrosurgical And Microsurgical Techniques In The Management Of The Tuboperitoneal Factor In Infertility. Fert Ster 32:377-383.

Siegler AM, Kontopoulos V, Wang CF (1980). Prevention Of Postoperative Adhesions In Rabbits With Ibuprofen, A Nonsteriodal Anti-Inflammatory Agent. Fert Ster 34:46-49.

Treatment of Post Surgical Adhesions, pages 23–33

ADHESION FORMATION/REFORMATION

Michael P. Diamond and Avner Hershlag

Department of Obstetrics & Gynecology, Division of Reproductive Endocrinology, Yale University School of Medicine, New Haven, CT 06510

The performance of adhesiolysis as a part of reproductive pelvic surgery is based on the premises that the extent and severity of pelvic adhesions can be reduced, and that such reduction will improve ultimate pregnancy outcome. Unfortunately, testing of these premises has been extremely limited, and the human studies which have been conducted are descriptive observations rather than well designed and controlled protocols. While awaiting better designed studies, the description that follows summarizes many of the reports available at this time.

The first premise is that adhesiolysis improves pregnancy outcome. While such reports are limited by the potential for coexisting infertility factors, they provide potential guidance for our patients. Bronson and Wallach (Bronson and Wallach, 1977) reported a 63% conception rate in 35 patients following adhesiolysis of periadnexal adhesions. In a larger series of 101 patients, Caspi et al (Caspi et al., 1979) reported conception in 39% following surgical adhesiolysis. They noted an inverse relationship between the extent of adhesions and the pregnancy rate. Jessen (Jessen, 1971) reported an improved pregnancy rate following lysis of adhesions in patients with low grade (64%) versus high grade (22%) adhesions. Hulka (Hulka, 1982) demonstrated that pregnancy was more likely to occur when over 50% of the ovary was visible, and when adhesions were filmy and avascular. These contentions have been challenged by other studies that will be discussed later on in this chapter.

It has been suggested that pelvic adhesions may impair fertility by interfering with ovum pickup by the tube, either by fixation of the ovary, fixation of the fallopian tube or encapsulation of these organs by adhesions thereby preventing the potential for pickup. A recent study on in vitro fertilization (IVF) patients has shown that periovarian adhesions do not compromise ovarian response to gonadotropin stimulation (Diamond et al., 1988). This finding supports the more commonly held opinion that the main mechanism by which pelvic adhesions impair fertility is impaired tubal function (eg ovum pickup) rather than interference in ovarian response.

Pregnancy outcome following adhesiolysis has a readily identified outcome, but its use as an end point of adhesiolysis is complicated by the myriad of coexisting factors which impair pregnancy outcome. A more direct end point to the efficacy of adhesiolysis is the ability to reduce adhesions. However, such documentation is not currently possible without performing a second invasive operative procedure. To be most accurate, such procedures would need to be performed shortly after the initial procedure and in a uniform manner to minimize the potential for confounding events due to either intercurrent pelvic processes, or selection bias as to which patients undergo a second-look procedure (eg only those who do not conceive).

Following reproductive pelvic surgical procedures, adhesions reform in 55-100% of women (Diamond, 1988). From studies with long term follow-up (eg years), it appears that the extent and severity of adhesions increases with the time that elapses from surgery (Diamond et al., 1984; DeCherney and Mezer, 1984; McLaughlin, 1984; Surrey and Friedman, 1982). In a multicenter study by Diamond et al (Diamond et al., 1987), adhesion reformation was evaluated in 121 women at early second-look laparoscopy (SLL). All women had undergone laparotomy for infertility utilizing the tenets of gynecologic microsurgery, surgical adjuvants, and the carbon dioxide laser. Of these women, 91 had a reduction in their total adhesion score, 16 had no change in the adhesion score, and in 14 the adhesion score increased. Adhesions reformed at one site or more where adhesions were initially identified and lysed surgically. The rate or type of adhesions reformed did not differ as a function of whether the initial adhesions were fine and filmy or dense and vascular. Lysis of organized, vascular adhesions did result in reduction in adhesion scores in the ovaries, fimbria and other locations. It thus seems, that contrary to previous contentions that vascular and dense adhesions carry a worse prognosis, adhesion reformation seems to be independent of the initial type of adhesion. In the same study, 51% of the patients were noticed on SLL to have developed de novo adhesions, that is, involvement of sites by adhesions at the time of SLL that were adhesion-free at the time of the initial procedure. In these women, such de novo adhesion formation developed at 31% of the available pelvic sites. Among these de novo adhesions, 82% were fine and filmy, while 18% were dense and vascular. Thus, it is overwhelmingly clear that reproductive pelvic surgery is all too frequently complicated by postoperative adhesion development, and that such adhesions represent not only adhesion reformation, but de novo adhesion formation as well.

Second-look laparoscopy

Second-look laparoscopy (SLL) has been utilized as a means of assessing the anatomic status of the pelvis after reproductive pelvic surgery. Such procedures provide a method of evaluating adhesion reformation or de novo formation, in addition to allowing another chance to lyse the adhesions. The timing of SLL reported in the literature has varied from 1 week to 3 years postoperatively (Diamond, 1988). Trimbos-Kemper et al. (Trimbos-Kemper et al., 1985) have reported early SLL and a "third look" laparoscopy one year later. Cumulative pregnancy rates were not improved, but in those women who underwent early SLL the extent of adhesions at the third look was reduced as was the rate of ectopic pregnancy. No controlled studies have been available yet to examine the influence of SLL on eventual pregnancy outcome. Until an alternate and preferably noninvasive method is available to evaluate for pelvic adhesion disease and tubal malfunction, performing early laparoscopy postoperatively seems to be a reasonable approach.

The use of the CO_2 laser

Both animal and human studies have somewhat "cooled off"

the initial laser-induced enthusiasm. In rabbits and rats, no reduction in post-operative adhesion was seen when the CO_2 laser was compared with fine needle cautery (Pittaway et al., 1983; Filmer et al., 1986). A multicenter prospective study in humans has shown, that while greater tubal patency was achieved using the CO_2 laser, as compared to non-laser surgery, adhesion prevention was not improved (Diamond et al., 1984; Adhesion Study Group, 1983). Varying success was shown of laser and non-laser techniques in preventing adhesions at different sites.

Adjuvants shown to reduce adhesion reformation Tables 1 & 2

TABLE: 1.

Proposed mechanisms of adhesion prevention by class of adjuvants

Class of Adjuvant	Proposed Mechanism
Antiinflammatory	Reduce vascular permeability, reduce histamine release and stabilize lysozomes
Progestins	Immunosuppression: decreased antibody production, inhibition of human mixed lymphocytic culture and leukocyte migration, decreased vascular permeability
Fibrinolytic enzymes	Fibrinolysis; stimulation of plasminogen activator
Antibiotics	Prevent infection
Mechanical separation	Surface separation, hydro floatation, siliconization

TABLE: 2.

Adjuvants found to be effective in the prevention of adhesion formation/reformation

AGENT	FORMATION		REFORMATION	
	ANIMALS	HUMANS	ANIMALS	HUMAN
Hyskon	Rabbits[1]	Adhesion Study Group[11]	Rabbits[14]	Adhesion Study Group[11]
		Rosenberg[12]		
	Monkeys[2]	Jessen[13]	Rabbits[15]	
CMC	Rabbits[3]		Rabbits[16]	
	Rats[4,5]		Rats[5]	
Calcium Channel Blockers	Hamsters[6,7]		Rabbits[17]	
Plasminogen Activator	Rabbits[8]		Rabbits[8]	
Interceed (TC-7)	Rabbits[9,10]			Interceed Study Group

1. Holtz et al., 1980.
2. DiZerga and Hodgen, 1980.
3. Diamond et al., 1988.
4. Elkins et al., 1984a.
5. Elkins et al., 1984b.
6. Steinleitner et al., 1988b.
7. Steinleitner et al., 1988a.
8. Doody et al., 1989.
9. Diamond et al., 1987.
10. Linsky et al., 1980.
11. Adhesion Study Group
12. Rosenberg and Board,1984.
13. Jessen, 1971.
14. Mazuji and Fadhi, 1965.
15. Holtz and Baker, 1980.
16. Diamond et al., 1988.
17. Steinleitner et al, 1989.

Mechanical separation of pelvic structures may be achieved either by intraabdominal instillates or barrier methods. High viscosity instillates are thought to work, at least in part, by third spacing of fluids into the abdominal cavity, creating an intraperitoneal "floatation bath." When this happens during the period of epithelial regeneration, apposition of serosal and peritoneal surfaces is limited, and adhesion formation is potentially reduced. The most widely studied adjuvant is Hyskon, or 32% Dextran 70 (molecular weight 70,000). In addition to the floatation effect, it is thought to prevent fibrin deposition (Mizaffar et al., 1972). Conflicting results have been obtained using Hyskon in experimental animals. Mazuji and Fadhli (Mazuji and Fadhi, 1965) found a large dose of dextran 75 (20 ml/kg of body weight) effective in inhibiting adhesion reformation. Since equivalent doses are not considered safe for use in humans, Holtz et al tried to repeat these experiments with lower doses of Hyskon. Using 2.5 ml/kg of body weight, Hyskon did not reduce adhesion reformation (Holtz et al., 1980). However, using higher doses of 5 ml/kg in one group of rabbits and 10 ml/kg in another, a significant inhibition of adhesion reformation was documented (Holtz and Baker, 1980). These studies seem to indicate that larger doses of Hyskon are needed to overcome adhesion reformation as compared with the initial lower dose which was successful in preventing adhesion formation. Whether this phenomenon points to a different mechanism, or whether factors leading to adhesion formation are operating at a larger scale with reformation, has not been elucidated. In a prospective, randomized, blinded, multicenter clinical trial, Hyskon significantly reduced adhesion formation, as observed by SLL, at the ovary, cul-de-sac and pelvic sidewall (Adhesion Study Group, 1983). No significant side effects of Hyskon were encountered in that report. A subsequent human study also demonstrated beneficial effects of 32% dextran 70. However two other human studies failed to identify any benefit of Hyskon in the reduction of postoperative adhesion development. However, the use of Hyskon has been restricted by many surgeons in recent years, perhaps due to these more recent human studies or possibly case reports of multiple side effects, including labial edema, fever, anaphylaxis, wound separation, shock, adult respiratory distress syndrome, serum sickness, disseminated intravascular coagulation, allergic peritonitis, pleural effusion, pseudopulmonary embolus, and hypokalemia (Holtz, 1985; Tulandi, 1987; Adoni et al., 1980; Ring and Messmer, 1977).

Another agent which has undergone evaluation as a potential adjuvant is sodium carboxymethylcellulose (CMC). CMC is prepared by reacting sodium monochloride with cellulose (Elkins et al., 1984). Theoretically it works by coating the intraperitoneal surface, thus preventing direct apposition of traumatized structure (Diamond et al., 1988). Its very slow absorption from the peritoneal cavity appears to be effective in producing a prolonged period for hydrofloatation thus potentially reducing postoperative adhesions (Elkins et al., 1984a). Elkins et al (Elkins et al., 1984b) found CMC to be effective in reducing adhesion reformation in rats, and that CMC was significantly more effective than 32% dextran 70 in the prevention of the reformation of adhesions. Fredericks et al (Fredericks et al., 1986) found CMC to be highly effective in reducing postoperative adhesions in the rabbit, in a dose-related fashion. Diamond et al (Diamond et al., 1988) found CMC to significantly reduce adhesion formation and reformation, using the rabbit uterine horn model.

More recently, calcium channel blocking agents (CCBA) such as verapamil, diltiazem and nifedipine have been used to prevent adhesion formation (Steinleitner et al., 1989; Steinleitner et al., 1988a; Steinleitner et al., 1988b). The hypothesis that such agents may help prevent adhesion formation is related to the role of calcium metabolism in the regulation of several of the cellular elements (eg fibroblasts, phagocytes, platelets and endothelial cells) involved in peritoneal repair. In the rabbit uterine horn model verapamil-treated animals formed significantly fewer adhesions following adhesiolysis than did controls (Steinleitner et al., 1989).

Tissue plasminogen activator (t-PA) converts plasminogen to plasmin. This activation occurs on the fibrin surface. Dissolution of fibrin then causes release of plasmin into the free circulation, where it is immediately bound and inactivated by antiplasmin. Topically applied recombinant t-PA (rt-PA) significantly reduced adhesion formation both in quantity and density, using the rabbit uterine horn model (Doody et al., 1989). Subsequently, rt-PA was shown to be an effective adjunct to surgical adhesiolysis in the same model (Doody et al., 1989). Adhesion reformation by rt-PA was reduced in a dose-related fashion.

Several kinds of barriers have been used to prevent adhesions. Oxidized cellulose (Surgicel) has decreased subsequent adhesion formation in several studies (Larrson et al., 1978; Raftery, 1980), while in another study adhesion development was enhanced (Hixon et al., 1986). Modifications of Surgicel (including degree of oxidation, density, porosity, and denier) have been developed, and named first TC-7 and later Interceed* TC-7 (Johnson and Johnson Patient Care). Rabbit studies have evaluated adhesion formation following use of Interceed* (TC-7) and demonstrated a significant reduction in adhesion scores in two rabbit models (Diamond et al., 1987; Linsky et al., 1987). In a later study, Interceed* (TC-7) was used in 74 women who had bilateral sidewall adhesions, with each woman acting as her own control. On SLL, the use of Interceed* (TC-7) had resulted in a significant reduction in the incidence of adhesion reformation (Interceed (TC-7) Barrier Study Group).

In conclusion, pelvic adhesions reform within a few days after surgery on the internal female genitalia. De novo adhesion formation has been described as well. Second look laparoscopy is the major existing means to diagnose and treat reformed and de novo formed adhesions. Although the pathogenesis of adhesion formation is complex and not fully understood at present, meticulous surgical technique is of value in reducing future adhesions. The use of lasers has not been found superior to alternative surgical techniques in reducing adhesion formation.

Although multiple adjuvants have been studied in relation to adhesion formation, only a few have been tested for adhesion reformation. Such animal studies have suggested that adjuvants are more effective in reducing adhesion formation than adhesion reformation. Explanation for this difference has not been elucidated; it may relate to alteration in the healing process in previously damaged (eg adhesed) tissues. A better understanding of the pathophysiology, perhaps at the molecular level, may promote future development in therapy. In addition, genetic engineering may allow us the use of recombinant forms of several compounds known to participate in the normal peritoneal healing process, thus allowing correction of abnormalities that may underlie adhesion formation and reformation.

REFERENCES

Adhesion Study Group (Buttram VC, Malinak R, Cleary R) (1983). Reduction of postoperative pelvic adhesions with intraperitoneal 32% Dextran 70: A prospective, randomized clinical trial. Fertil Steril 40: 612-619.

Adoni A, Adatto-Levi R, Mogle P (1980). Post-operative pleural effusion caused by dextran. Int J Gynecol Obstet 18: 243.

Bronson RA, Wallach EE (1977). Lysis of periadnexal adhesion for correction of infertility. Fertil Steril 26: 613-619.

Caspi E, Halperin Y, Bukovsky I (1979). The importance of periadnexal adhesion in tubal reconstructive surgery for infertility. Fertil Steril 31: 296-300.

DeCherney AH, Mezer HC (1984). The nature of posttuboplasty pelvic adhesions as determined by early and late laparoscopy. Fertil Steril 41: 643.

Diamond MP, Linsky CB, Cunningham T, et al (1988). Assessment of carboxymethylcellulose and 32% dextran 70 for prevention of adhesions in a rabbit uterine horn model. Int J Fertil 33: 278.

Diamond MP, Daniell JF, Feste J et al (1987). Adhesion reformation and de noro adhesion formation after reproductive pelvic surgery. Fertil Steril 47: 864-866.

Diamond MP, Daniell JF, Feste J, et al (1984). Pelvic adhesions at second look laparoscopy following carbon dioxide laser surgery procedures. Infertility 7: 39.

Diamond MP (1988). Surgical Aspects of Infertility. In: Sciarra, 61: 1-23.

Diamond MP, Daniell JF, Martin DC et al (1984). Tubal patency and pelvic adhesions at early second look laparoscopy following intraabdominal use of carbon dioxide laser: Initial report of the intraabdominal laser study group. Fertil Steril 42: 717-723.

Diamond MP, Pellicer A, Boyers SP (1988). The effect of periovarian adhesion of follicular development in patients undergoing ovarian stimulation for in vitro fertilization-embryo transfer. Fertil Steril 49: 100-103.

Diamond MP, Linsky CB, Cunningham T et al (1987). A model for sidewall adhesion in the rabbit: Reduction by an absorbable barrier. Microsurgery 8: 197-200.

Diamond MP, DeCherney AH, Linsky CB, Cunningham T, Constantine B (1988). Adhesion Re-formation in the rabbit uterine horn model: 1. Reduction with carboxymethyl cellulose. Int J Infertil 33: 372-735.

DiZerega GS, Hodgen GD (1980). Prevention of postoperative tubal adhesions. Am J Obstet Gynecol 136: 173-178.

Doody KJ, Dunn RC, Buttram VC (1989). Recombinant tissue plasminogen activator reduces adhesion formation in a rabbit uterine horn model. Fertil Steril 51: 509.

Elkins TE, Bury RJ, Ritter JL et al (1984a). Adhesion prevention by solutions of sodium carboxymethyl cellulose in the rat, I. Fertil Steril 41: 926-928.

Elkins TE, Ling FW, Ahokas RA et al (1984b). Adhesion prevention by solution of sodium carboxymethyl cellulose in the rat, II. Fertil Steril 41: 929-932.

Filmer S, Gomel V, McComb P (1986). The effectiveness of CO_2 laser and electromicrosurgery adhesiolysis: A comparative study. Fertil Steril 45: 407.

Fredericks CM, Kotry I, Holtz G et al. (1986). Adhesion prevention in the rabbit with sodium carboxymethylcellulose solutions. Am J Obstet Gynecol 155: 667.

Hixon C, Swanson LA, Friedman CI (1986). Oxidized cellulose for preventing adnexal adhesions. J Reprod Med 311: 58-60.

Holtz G, Baker E, Tasi C (1980). Effect of thirty-two percent Dextran 70 on peritoneal adhesion formation and re-formation after lysis. Fertil Steril 33: 660.

Holtz G (1985). Current use of ancillary modalities for adhesion formation. Fertil Steril 44: 174-176.

Holtz G, Baker ER (1980). Inhibition of peritoneal adhesion reformation after lysis with thirty-two percent Dextran 70. Fertil Steril 34: 394-395.

Hulka JF (1982). Adnexal adhesions: A prognostic staging and classification system based on a five-year survey of fertility surgery results at Chapel Hill, North Carolina. Am J Obstet Gynecol 144: 141.

Interceed (TC-7) Barrier Study Group (1989). Prevention of post-surgical adhesions by Interceed (TC-7), an absorbable adhesion barrier: A prospective randomized multicenter clinical study. Fertil Steril 51: 933.

Jessen H (1971). Operations for sterility. Acta Obstet Gynecol Scand 50: 105.

Larsson B, Nisell H, Grandberg I (1978). Surgicel - an absorbable hemostatic material in prevention of peritoneal adhesions in rats. Acta Chir Scand 144: 375.

Linsky CB, Diamond MP, Cunningham T et al (1987). Adhesion reduction in the rabbit uterine horn model using an absorbable barrier, TC-7. J Reprod Med 32: 17-20.

Mazuji MK, Fadhi HA (1965). Peritoneal adhesions. ARch Surg 91: 872.

McLaughlin DS (1984). Evaluation of adhesion reformation by early second look laparoscopy following microlaser ovarian wedge resection. Fertil Steril 42: 531.

Mizaffar TZ, Youngson GG, Bryce WAJ, Hall DP (1972). Studies on fibrin formation of effects of dextran. Thromb Diath Hemorrh 28: 244.

Pittaway DE, Maxon WS, Daniell JF (1983). A comparison of the CO_2 laser and electrocautery on postoperative intraperitoneal adhesion formation in rabbits. Fertil Steril 40: 366.

Raftery A (1980). Absorbable hemostatic materials and intraperitoneal adhesion formation. Br J Surg 67: 57.

Ring J, Messmer K (1977). Incidence and severity of anaphylactoid reaction to colloid volume substitutes. Lancet 1:446.

Rosenberg SM, Board JA (1984). High-molecular weight dextran in human infertility surgery. Am J Obstet Gynecol 148: 380.

Steinleitner A, Lambert H, Montoro L et al (1988a). The use of calcium channel blockade for the prevention of postoperative adhesion formation. Fertil Steril 50: 818.

Steinleitner A, Lambert H, Montoro L, Swanson J, Sueldo CE (1988b). Use of diltiozem for preventing postoperative adhesions. J Reprod Med 33: 891.

Steinleitner A, Kozensky C, Lambert H (1989). Calcium channel blockade prevents adhesion reformation following adhesiolysis (Abstract). Presented at the 37th Annual Clinical Meeting of the American College of Surgeons in Atlanta, May 1989.

Surrey MW, Friedman S (1982). Second look laparoscopy after reconstructive pelvic surgery for infertility. J Reprod Med 27: 658.

Trimbos-Kemper TCM, Trimbos JB, van Hall EV: Adhesion formation after tubal surgery: Results of the eighth day laparoscopy in 188 patients. Fertil Steril 43:395, 1985.

Tulandi T (1987). Transient edema after intraperitoneal instillation of 32% Dextran 70: A report of five cases. J Reprod Med 32: 472-474.

Treatment of Post Surgical Adhesions, pages 35–44

LAPAROTOMY VERSUS LAPAROSCOPY

Anthony A. Luciano M.D.
Associate Professor of Obstetrics and Gynecology, Director of Reproductive Endocrinology, University of Connecticut School of Medicine, Farmington, Connecticut 06032

Besides the severity of pre-existing disease, the major determinants of the outcome of infertility surgery are postoperative adhesion formation and the extent of tissue injury at and beyond the surface of the wound (Ellis 1971; Bronson and Wallach, 1977; Caspi et al., 1979; Weinstein and Polishuk, 1975). To minimize the extent of tissue injury and the formation of peritoneal adhesions, medical adjuvants and improved surgical techniques have been introduced to the armamentarium of the reproductive surgeon. Although no adjuvant has thus far enjoyed lasting success, the discipline of microsurgery has stood the test of time and represents a major contribution to the current success of reproductive surgery (Gomel and McComb, 1975).

Microsurgery connotes not only the use of magnification but the whole concept of fine surgery which embodies the discipline of gentle handling of tissues, constant irrigation, meticulous hemostasis, the use of microsurgical instruments, fine sutures (when necessary), and precise tissue dissection and approximation. Still, we continue to be faced with too many failures (Gomel and McComb, 1979; Swolin, 1975; Carey and Brown, 1987) and the search for better techniques continues.

During the past decade, we have witnessed the emergence of operative endoscopy and laser surgery in the hope of providing our infertile women with better pregnancy rates. Although useful and versatile, lasers do not seem to have significant advantages over the more traditional microsurgical or electrosurgical tools (Luciano et al., 1987; and Filmar et al., 1989). More promising however appears to be the discipline of endoscopic surgery (DeCherney, 1985) which fulfills the most important criteria of microsurgery, as outlined above, without the need for laparotomy which is in itself a significant invasion of the peritoneal cavity.

The recognized advantages of endoscopic surgery over laparotomy include the obvious ones of convenience, quick recovery, and significant cost savings (DeCherney, 1985) But the most important goals of reconstructive pelvic surgery, results and success rates have not been adequately addressed in clinical studies.

Indeed, controlled studies comparing results from endoscopic versus laparotomy surgery with similar procedures performed by the same surgeon have not been done and may be difficult to carry out. It may be considered unethical to randomize patients to the more invasive and significantly more expensive laparotomy procedure. Thus, one must resort to animal studies which can be randomized and properly controlled. Recently, we carried out such studies in the rabbit model, comparing operative laser laparoscopy versus laparotomy in postoperative adhesion formation and reduction following a standardized laser injury and adhesiolysis (Luciano et al., 1989).

Methodology. Twenty rabbits were randomly assigned to either laparoscopy or laparotomy and subjected to standardized laser incision over one uterine horn and over the peritoneal surface of either lower quadrant. Three weeks later, 5 animals from each group underwent laparoscopy and the other 5 laparotomy to score the extent of postoperative adhesions formed and to carry out laser adhesiolysis. To ascertain that comparable tissue injuries were inflicted by both surgical procedures, after measuring the spot size the laser wattage was adjusted so that the same power density was delivered to tissues in both laparoscopy and laparotomy. Three weeks after the second operative intervention, the animals were killed and the intraperitoneal adhesions reassessed and scored (scale: 0-3). Thus the laparoscopic and open abdominal procedures were compared after standard surgical trauma and after adhesiolysis, as illustrated in the following diagram:

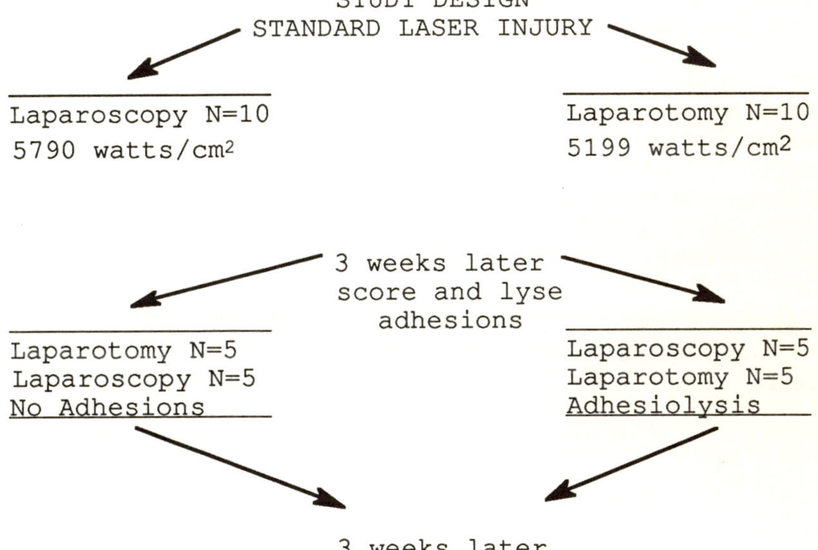

In these experiments we wished to: 1) compare postoperative adhesion formation following a standardized laser injury by laparoscopy versus laparotomy; 2) evaluate postoperative adhesion formation on tissues which were not directly involved in the surgical lesions; and 3) evaluate and compare adhesion reduction following adhesiolysis by laser laparoscopy versus laparotomy.

Following the initial surgical procedure, when standardized laser injuries were carried out on the uterine horn and peritoneal surface of the anterior abdominal wall, adhesions were present in every rabbit that had undergone laparotomy but were totally absent in the laparoscopy group. In this latter group, the injury on the peritoneal surface of the abdominal wall was completely healed, with deposition of new peritoneum without evidence of scar tissue. In eight of these animals, the operated uterine horn appeared so normal that we could not discern which side had been ablated. In 2 animals, the horn was narrow or partially obliterated but had no adhesions. In the laparotomy group, adhesions were frequently present not only at the sites of injury and on the peritoneal surface of the abdominal wall where the laparotomy incision was made, but also on the opposite uterine horn, bowel and bladder, where no apparent injury had been inflicted. The table below summarizes the results of postoperative adhesion formation at the sites of the initial injury and at other sites.

Table 1. Mean (±SD) Postoperative Adhesion Scores Following Standard Injury With CO_2 Laser By Laparoscopy Versus Laparotomy

	Horn	Sidewall	Incidental
Laparoscopy	0	0	0
Laparotomy	1.7±.4	2.1±.3	1.2±.4
P= (Wilcoxon signed test)	0.009	0.004	0.02

The 10 animals that had undergone initial laparotomy underwent extensive adhesiolysis by laparoscopy in 5 and by laparotomy in the other 5, using the CO2 laser at the same, comparable power densities as for the standardized injuries. Three weeks after adhesiolysis, when the animals were killed and the final adhesions were scored, the mean postoperative adhesion scores were significantly reduced in the laparoscopy but not in the laparotomy group as shown in the following Figure.

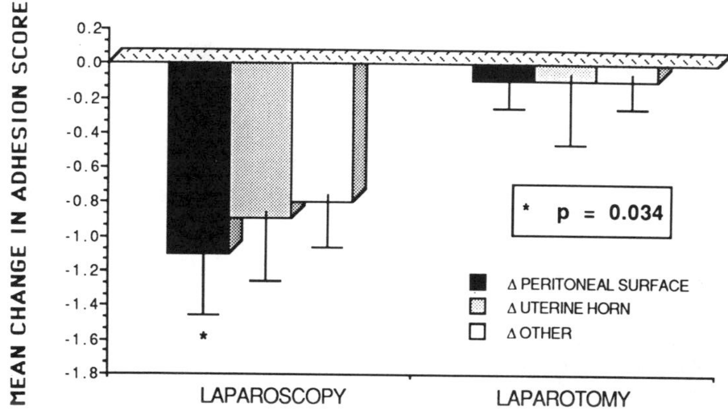

Figure 1. Changes in the mean (± SEM) postoperative adhesion scores at the surgical and incidental sites following laser adhesiolysis by labaroscopy versus laparotomy.

Because endoscopic surgery is carried out from a distance, the laser beam is ideally suited for this technique. Therefore, although the advantages of laser over standard microsurgery and electrosurgery have not been documented in open abdominal procedures (Luciano et al., 1987 and Filmar et al., 1989), in laparoscopic surgery the laser may be advantageous because It can be directed to all areas of the peritoneal cavity and, by using varying power densities, one may excise, ablate, or coagulate superficial or deep structures as needed.

Because it can be easily delivered from a distance, the laser is ideally suited for the laparoscope which provides magnification with excellent exposure and access to all areas of the peritoneal cavity. Moreover, laparoscopy involves minimal manipulation of target tissues and surrounding structures, and it allows the procedure to be performed in a closed system (the abdomen is not open) so that the peritoneal organs are not exposed to the atmosphere, minimizing the potential for not only infections but also dryness of the peritoneal surfaces which predisposes to adhesion formation (Ryan et al, 1971).

Our comparative study demonstrates a major advantage of endoscopic surgery over laparotomy in postoperative adhesion formation after a standard laser injury to the intraperitoneal organs (Luciano et al., 1989). Indeed, in the laparotomy group postoperative adhesions were present not only on the tissues directly involved with the initial injury (uterine horn and peritoneal surface of the abdominal wall), but also on other peritoneal surfaces which were not touched by the laser. The formation of incidental (de novo) adhesions following laparotomy, are consistent with the findings of Diamond et al., 1987 who reported that "de novo adhesions developed at at least one location in 51% of cases" of women who had undergone pelvic laser adhesiolysis by laparotomy (Diamond et al., 1987). In our study, de novo adhesions did not occur after laparoscopic surgery (table 1).

Similar observations have recently been noted by Nezhat et al., following a second look laparoscopy in 157 patients who had undergone initial videolaseroscopy for the treatment of endometriosis-associated infertility. In this report, videolaseroscopy effectively reduced peritoneal adhesions and was devoid of de novo adhesion formation (Nezhat et al., 1989).

Besides our study, the only other study that compared operative laparoscopy with laparotomy for postoperative adhesion formation was by Filmar et al., who inflicted a standard injury with sharp scissors on the uterine horn of rabbits (Filmar et al., 1987). These investigators reported no significant difference between the two procedures in postoperative adhesion formation. The difference from our results may be explained in that Filmar et al. inflicted the injury on the uterine horn with sharp scissors, which they stated resulted in "bleeding in every instance... which was not immediately controlled." In our experience with animal studies, especially rats, the most severe adhesions occur after open abdominal procedures that are complicated by significant bleeding (Ryan et al., 1971 and Luciano et al., 1983). In the current study, when bleeding occurred, it was immediately controlled by the laser beam using either operative technique.

Although the results from standardized injuries are useful in that they satisfy the criteria for randomization and controls, these studies do not truly reflect the clinical situation in which reconstructive pelvic surgery is performed on tissues that have suffered injury and have healed with deposition of scars that distort the anatomy and impede function. Therefore, the results from our second operative procedure become much more meaningful, and from them we can better assess and compare the efficacy of reconstructive laser surgery performed by laparoscopy versus laparotomy. When we consider the changes in the adhesion scores before to after adhesiolysis (Figure 1) a significant reduction occurred in the laparoscopy but not in the laparotomy group.

From the studies in the literature on the evaluation of postoperative adhesion formation after laparotomy, we may conclude that reproductive pelvic surgery procedures are frequently complicated not only by adhesion formation but also by *de novo* adhesion formation (Diamond et al., 1989; Trimbos-Kemper et al., 1985; McLaughlin, 1983). Following microsurgical salpingoplasty, Trimbos-Kemper et al., found that adhesions were present in more than 50% of the cases, when evaluated on the 8th postoperative day (Trimbos-Kemper et al., 1985). Similarly, using microlaser techniques, recurrence of adnexal adhesions occurred in 40%-72% of cases (Diamond et al., 1987 and McLaughlin, 1983). The results from our animal studies and a recent report from Nezhat et al. on the clinical experience in patients with endometriosis (Luciano et al., 1989 and Nezhat et al., 1989) suggest that when comparable extensive surgical procedures are performed by laparoscopy, the recurrence of intraperitoneal adhesions may be significantly lower than when performed by laparotomy.

The data from this study confirm the clinical impression that postoperative adhesion formation is uncommon following operative laparoscopic surgery (Filmar et al., 1989) and suggest a possible explanation why for the more severe and extensive stages of endometriosis, operative laser laparoscopy is associated with better pregnancy rates and higher fecundity rates than those reported following laparotomy (Olive and Martin, 1983 and Nezhat et al., 1989). It is now becoming quite clear, that in experienced hands, operative laparoscopy should be preferred to the more traditional microsurgical approach of laparotomy in the treatment of most benign gynecologic surgical procedures.

REFERENCES

Bronson RA, Wallach EE (1977). Lysis of periadnexal adhesions for correction of infertility. Fertil Steril 28:613-617.

Carey M, Brown S (1987). Infertility surgery for pelvic inflammatory disease: success rates after salpingolysis and salpingostomy. Am J Obstet Gynecol 156:296-300.

Caspi E, Halperin Y, Bukawsky J (1979). The importance of periadnexal adhesions in tubal reconstructive surgery for infertility. Fertil Steril 31:296-298.

Ellis H (1971). The cause and prevention of postoperative intraperitoneal adhesions. Surg Gynecol Obstet 133:497-511.

DeCherney AH (1985). The leader of the band is tired-. Fertil Steril 44:299-302.

Diamond MP, Daniell SF, Feste J, Surrey MW, McLaughlin DS, Friedman S, Vaughn WK, Martin DC (1987). Adhesion reformation and de novo adhesion formation after reproductive pelvic surgery. Fertil Steril 47:864-866.

Filmar S, Gomel V, McComb PF (1987). Operative laparoscopy versus open abdominal surgery: a comparative study on postoperative adhesion formation in the rat model. Fertil Steril 48:486-489.

Filmar S, Jetha N, McComb P, Gomel V (1989). A comparative histologic study on the healing process after tissue transection I. Carbon dioxide laser and electromicrosurgery, II. Carbon dioxide laser and surgical microscissors. Am J Obstet Gynecol 160: 1062-72.

Gomel V, McComb P (1979). Microsurgery in Gynecology. In Microsurgery, (ed) Silver JS, Williams and Wilkins, Baltimore, Maryland 143-183.

Luciano AA, Hauser KS, Benda J (1983). Evaluation of commonly used adjuvants in the prevention of postoperative adhesions. Am J Obstet Gynecol 146:88-92.

Luciano AA, Maier DB, Koch EI, Nulsen JC, Whitman GF (1989). A comparative study of postoperative adhesions following laser surgery by laparoscopy versus laparotomy in the rabbit model. Obstet Gynecol 74:220-224.

Luciano AA, Whitman G, Maier DB, Randolph J, Maenza R (1987). A comparison of thermal injury, healing patterns, and postoperative adhesion formation following CO2 laser and electromicrosurgery. Fertil Steril 48:1025-9.

McLaughlin DS (1983). Evaluation of adhesion reformation by early second-look laparoscopy following microlaser ovarian wedge resection. Fertil Steril 42:531-537.

Nezhat C, Crowgey S, Nezhat F (1989). Videolaseroscopy for the treatment of endometriosis associated infertility. Fertil Steril 51:237-240.

Nezhat C, Nezhat F, Luciano AA (1989). Adhesion reformation following reproductive surgery by videolaseroscopy. Fertil Steril. Submitted for publication.

Olive DL, Martin DC (1987). Treatment of endometriosis-associated infertility with CO_2 laser laparoscopy: the use of 1- and 2-parameter exponential models. Fertil Steril 48:18-23.

Ryan GB, Grobety J, Majno G. Postoperative peritoneal adhesions (1971). Am J Pathol 65:117-48.

Swolin K (1975). Electromicrosurgery and salpingostomy - long-term results. Am J Obstet Gynecol 121:418-422.

Trimbos-Kemper TCM, Trimbos JB, van Hall EV (1985). Adhesion formation after tubal surgery: results of the eight day laparoscopy in 188 patients. Fertil Steril 43:395.

Weinstein D, Polishuk WZ (1975). The role of wedge resection of the ovary as a cause for mechanical sterility. Surg Gynecol Obstet 141:41-421.

Treatment of Post-Surgical Adhesions, pages 45–58

MICROSURGICAL ADHESIOLYSIS

Carl J. Levinson, M.D.
Clinical Professor Department of Obstetrics, Gynecology & Reproductive SciencesUniversity of California San Francisco,
Chairman of the Department of Obstetrics & Gynecology, Children's Hospital San Francisco

INTRODUCTION AND OVERVIEW

Adhesions are the bete noire of tubal and ovarian surgery, particularly true following the painstaking skills and care required for proper microsurgery. If microsurgical techniques (in the fullest sense) were to be successful, postoperative adhesions would not occur. However, they do and present a formidable problem, particularly in problems of infertility. Adhesions may close the Fallopian Tube, coat the ovary and interfere with the mechanics of ovulation, distort tubal relationships, interfere with ovum pick-up by the tube, adhere foreign structures (e.g. omentum and bowel) to the pelvic organs, fix the uterus in abnormal position and distort any and all pelvic relationships. The adhesions may be filmy and veil-like or thick, vascular and fibrous. The extent to which adhesions within the pelvis interfere with the processes leading to fertilization and implantation depend on a variety of factors: etiology, location, extent, duration, thickness, vascularity and structures involved.

This paper shall limit itself to the subject of "adhesions" as it relates to microsurgical techniques.

CHARACTERISTICS OF MICROSURGICAL "TECHNIQUE"

In reality, microsurgical "techniques" have all the same characteristics outlined by Halstead plus the use of optics to enlarge and better define tissue planes. Magnification (best by microscope, improved by loupes) allows for better observation, dissection and approximation. Lavage of the tissue with physiologic solution keeps the field clear while eliminating the trauma of sponging. The use of electrosurgical or laser techniques for dissection provide pinpoint hemostasis, thereby replacing the clamp-tie-cut technique. Fine suture material with appropriate-sized needle results in minimal tissue reaction. Wherever possible, raw surfaces are eliminated by careful reperitonealization. The handling of tissue is minimized. Overall, the microsurgical approach emphasizes excellent visibility, gentle tissue handling and meticulous attention to the surgical principles of hemostasis, dissection and approximation of tissue.

ETIOLOGY
PHYSIOLOGY

The etiologic factors involved in adhesion formation and the physiology of the reparative processes of tissues are found in another section.

PREOPERATIVE ASPECTS

During the 1970's there was a marked incremental use of microsurgical techniques in Gynecology. Along with the specific use of magnification, there was an increased interest in the use of ancillary techniques for adhesion prevention. All have a rationale but controlled prospective studies are rare. Some valid information is available, augmented by the prospect of greater numbers and longer follow-up so that a more intelligent "clinical" (if not scientific) evaluation is possible.

Selection of Patients: A candid approach would indicate that most patients do the selecting, not the surgeon. It is incumbent upon the physician to assess the situation: history, all records, physical examination, HSG and laparoscopy. Once these have been gathered, determination regarding the suitability of microsurgery (plus a broad prognostic assessment) can be determined. In the 1970's, the "microsurgical" approach appeared to be the most sophisticated in assisting of a couple seeking infertility related to adhesions. In the 1980's, this concept was challenged by the advent of In Vitro Fertilization and the extended possibility of performing the same surgery by endoscopic techniques. Laparoscopy and/or HSG were performed for preoperative evaluation. The surgical procedure was generally carried out in the immediate post-menstrual phase. Very often, laparoscopy was performed initially with a microsurgical technique to follow under the same anesthesia, if appropriate.

Preoperative Medication: Prophylactic antibiotics are commonly used but are by no means universal. They are most likely to be given to those patients whose disease process results from a prior infection. Doxycycline commonly employed in view of reports of the increasing incidence of Chlamydia. The primary rationale is the fear of postoperative pelvic infection. Such infections are rare; no controlled studies exist in the literature. Steroids, at one time recommended for preoperative use, are rarely utilized at this time.

INTRA-OPERATIVE ASPECTS

Positioning of the Patient: The patient should be comfortably located on the table, either in the supine position or the "frog leg" position, according to the choice of the surgeon. The arms are best located alongside the patient so as to allow for appropriate physician mobility.

Use of Intrauterine Catheter: A variety of methods have been used. Probably the most common is the use of a flexible plastic catheter with a balloon to be located within the uterine cavity and a plastic disc at the external cervix. This is then connected to tubing, extending to a syringe filled with diluted indigo carmine. This latter is taped to the lateral end of the table so that it can be controlled by either an assistant or the circulating nurse.

<u>Position of the Operator</u>: The surgeon may stand or sit, a matter of personal preference. Microsurgical procedures do not last 6-8 hours and 3-4 hours is unusual. In any event, the operator must adjust the microscope height so as to be comfortably erect. The use of back braces and hand rests are individual matters. If the surgeon chooses to sit, the operating table must have room beneath for the surgeon's knees. Comfort and the minimization of fatigue are the bywords.

<u>Removal of Talc:</u> Nowhere is it more significant to be certain that all powder and talc are removed from the surgical gloves prior to the incision. These have been well documented to develop granulomata within the body.

<u>Incision:</u> The incision is a matter of choice, and to some degree, patient desire. A vertical incision is easier, quicker and provides more room. However, a low transverse incision is cosmetically desireable and more comfortable postoperatively. Almost universally, the Pfannenstiel incision is acceptable, providing good exposure of the pelvic organs.

<u>Mobilization and Elevation:</u> Some surgeons recommend packing of the vagina but this is not universally used. Whereas such packing may elevate the pelvic organs bringing them closer to the surface, in some instances the opposite result is obtained with fixation of the uterus and inhibition of mobility in the operative area. The same result may be obtained by intra-abdominal packing into the cul-de-sac (when freed), thereby providing good elevation of the adnexae and a platform on which adnexae may rest during the procedure. On rare occasions, a suture may be placed through the fundus and used to elevate the uterus or to bring it laterally.

<u>Irrigation</u>: Lavage is much preferable to

sponging: it is less traumatic and equally effective. The most physiologic solution readily available is Ringers Lactate. The cooling of fluid to room temperature during a 2-3 hour procedure is a problem which can be overcome by a blood warmer placed around the intravenous container. A number of techniques for lavage have been successful: irrigators with fingertip control attached to the solution elevated in a container or bulb syringes with plastic tips (which require frequent refilling).

Various medications have been added to the solution. the addition of heparin (2000-5000 i.u. per liter) has proven to be a great asset in that small clots are dissolved and large clots do not form. The mucosal and serosal surfaces are kept clean and smooth, presumably inhibiting adhesion formation.

Stents, Splints and Hoods: The use of any form of splint or covering has diminished markedly. Intra-lumenal splints have been shown to diminish mucosal viability and to destroy cilia. Short term splinting of the cornual area following tubal cornual anastomosis is frequently done. Hoods are available, made of extremely inert and delicate material. These coverings are placed over the repaired distal end of the tube to prevent adhesion formation to that site. Only a few operators currently use such hoods since there is no statistical evidence that the results are better and a second operation for removal is mandatory.

Unrelated Surgery: Most operators prefer to avoid additional unrelated surgery in that they tend to additional risk for adhesion formation. A specific example of this is myomectomy. Many surgeons prefer to do appendectomies as a prophylactic measure.

Prevention of Trauma: We have already referred to the gentle handling of tissue, preferably without the use of metallic instruments and such things as good approximation of tissue, minimal blood loss, prevention of desiccation of tissue, use of non-woven swabs and attention to the overall technique. Everyone has an old Department Chairman who had very special sayings to remember. Mine (Henry C. Falk, M.D.) used to say: "The best postoperative care is a good operation."

Suture Material: Although there is some controversy in this area, it is generally considered that the newer synthetic sutures are less likely to develop adhesions. However it is not clear whether the absorbable sutures are any different in this aspect from the non-absorbable sutures.

Intraperitoneal Medication: Although an early paper indicated that there might be benefit from the use of intraperitoneal cortisone, this agent is rarely used in this manner. Heparin is often added to the physiologic solution utilized for lavage in order to prevent the formation of blood clots. This is done by the inhibition of the formation of a fibrin matrix.

Systemic Medication: Early experimental work by Repogle demonstrated an inhibition of adhesion formation in dogs by the use of high doses of dexamethasone and promethazine. There was the necessity of large pharmacologic doses and a high level of saturation at the time of injury. Subsequently the results were borne out clinically in Pediatric surgical patients. Glucocorticoids reduce inflammatory exudate, stabilize the cell membrane and thereby protect against increased permeability and limits secondary inflammatory damage by inhibiting fibroblast proliferation and organization. The exact mechanism for the use of promethazine is unknown but it presumably acts as an antihistamine. The drug minimizes early inflammatory reaction and inhibits the histamine response, thereby lessening vascular permeability. It may also protect the cell lysozyme system.

Mechanical Separation of Surfaces: A wide variety of substances have been used over the years in an attempt to prevent adhesion formation by keeping raw peritoneal surfaces separated from each other as well as mucosal surfaces. As already indicated, splints placed within mucosal surfaces have negative effects on the endosalpinx, however inert the material. Various forms of plastic inert substances have been employed to cover the distal end of the tube following repair. These generally result in adhesion formation between the device and the serosa and require a second operative procedure for removal. They are no longer currently in wide use. Similarly, there has been extensive interest in the installation of high colloidal pressure fluids for the purpose of separating the surfaces of raw areas. Experimental and clinical results with all of these substances has been equivocal. Of these, high molecular dextran has been the most commonly utilized. It is a branched-chain polysaccharide. When placed within the peritoneal cavity, it induces transudation of serum into the peritoneal cavity. Dextran may result in the osmosis of 3-4 times its own quantity in fluid and may remain within the peritoneal cavity as long as 7-10 days. If large quantities are utilized, electrolyte balance must be carefully observed. Once again, both animal experiments and clinical observations have been equivocal.

POST OPERATIVE ASPECTS

Antibiotics: The use of prophylactic antibiotics has already been discussed. The practice is widespread although scientific support for such use is lacking.

Corticosteroids and Promethazine: The basis for the use of these substances has already been discussed. One cooperative clinical study indicated a significantly higher subsequent pregnancy rate for distal tubal disease when these substances were utilized. However, the study has never been repeated.

Hydrotubation: Over many decades, hydrotubation has been utilized as a means of establishing (or developing) patency of the Fallopian Tube. At one time it was considered an approach to open blocked tubes by forcing fluids through them. Today it is no longer utilized. It is questionable that it even serves a cleansing purpose: to remove debris and blood clots immediately postoperatively in cases of distal tubal surgery. No controlled studies are available although an early work indicated improved results in salpingostomy by performing early hydrotubation. In addition to being inconvenient, the passage of fluid through the cervix into the Fallopian Tubes and peritoneal cavity certainly increases the possibility of infection.

"Second-Look Laparoscopy": It has been proposed that a Second-Look Laparoscopy be performed, primarily for patients operated on for distal tubal disease due to inflammation. The primary purpose is the determination of recurrent adhesions and the possibility of lysing such adhesions. Timing has been variably reported from 8 days to 12 weeks postoperative. The author has a personal series of 120 cases following salpingostomy with the finding that 65% had recurrent adhesion formation. Lysing of the adhesions did not measurably increase the subsequent pregnancy rate. Although reports have been varied, this appears to be the common experience among microsurgeons.

EXPERIMENTAL DATA (RELATED TO MICROSURGERY)

Trauma: Swollin (1974) reported on a study in rats in which the peritoneum was stroked with woven swab (short cotton fibers), resulting in adhesions in 60%. When a non-woven swab was used (pure cellulose fibers), adhesions resulted in only 16.7%.

Antibiotics: Studies available are non-controlled and, in many instances, a report with many confounding factors.

Solution for Lavage: Blandau , working with laboratory animals observed edema in tissues submerged in normal saline whereas this situation was corrected if the tissues were placed in balanced salt solution.

Suture and Needle: A number of studies have shown that cat gut suture induces more inflammatory response than non-absorbable or synthetic absorbable sutures. Smith compared 10-0 Dermalon and 8-0 Vicryl sutures. The inflammatory response was approximately the same at 4 weeks but, at 6 months, there was lesser inflammatory reaction with Vicryl.

Prostheses and Splints: Winston has demonstrated that the presence of splints over a 4 week period results in a marked inflammatory reaction of the endosalpinx with fibrosis of the wall. In a clinical study, Wheeless could show excellent tubal patency following anastomosis but a very low pregnancy rate where a splint had been left within the tube for 3 months. Although there have been numerous reports regarding the use of "hoods" to cover the repaired distal end of the tube, there have been no controlled studies and the procedure is not generally utilized by those employing microsurgical techniques.

Steroids, Intraperitoneal: Swolin reported in 1967 on a series of laparotomies for ectopic pregnancy in which patients were treated equally except that half received an installation of intra-peritoneal hydrocortisone while the other half received saline. At Second Look Laparoscopy, the treated patients had fewer adhesions. A number of other studies have been performed, non-controlled, with confounding factors (use of antibiotics, parenteral corticoids, etc.) which show no such clear cut value to the use of glucocorticoids intraperitoneally.

Peritoneal Separation: The most commonly used agent is 32% dextran 70 in dextrose (Hyskon). The Adhesion Study Group (1983) performed a prospective randomized study in patients in which Hyskon 250 cc was instilled into the pelvis at the time of closure. When compared to patients who received saline, Dextran significantly reduced adhesions in those patients who originally had severe adnexal disease, A similar result was reported by Rosenberg and Board (1984). However, in both situations there were confounding factors (differences in surgical technique, variability of sutures, etc.) so that the results are difficult to assess. In a broad overview of the experimental animal literature as well as clinical results, there are numerous conflicting results as to the efficacy of Dextran...and no well controlled "relatively pure" studies.

Steroids, Systemic: Glucocorticoids are most commonly used for adhesion prevention, largely based on the study by Replogle et al in 1966. The steroids are most commonly administered in conjunction with antihistamines. A study by Liao et al in 1973 reported a diminution of adhesions using systemic steroids and antihistaminics while Seitz (1973) and di Zerega and Hodgen (1980) failed to show any effects at all. A single large study by Horne and co-workers (1973) utilized systemic Dexamethasone and Promethazine prior to and following surgery and reported an increase of clinical pregnancies in those patients having surgery for distal tube disease.

Antihistamines: These agents have been used almost uniformly in conjunction with the corticosteroids, described above.

Hydrotubation: A study by Grant (1971) reported a greater pregnancy rate (41%) when hydrotubation was repeated post-operatively, when compared to a preceding series of patients in whom it was not performed (16%). Subsequently Rock et al (1978) reported on a series of salpingostomy cases where the use of hydrotubation did not increase the frequency of pregnancy: this study was non-randomized.

RESULTS

Microscopic Adhesiolysis

There is great difficulty in determining the results of surgical procedures for infertility. Many factors influence the success rate. The criteria for selection of patients may differ. Some papers consider delivery of a patient on two separate occasions as a single success, others as two successes. There is no uniform definition of the "technique", particularly difficult in defining "fimbrioplasty" as compared to "salingo-ovariolysis". Since two tubes are often involved, there is often a variation in selection of one tube or both tubes. Certain technical and anatomical features are significant: the duration of the disease process; duration of the procedure; extent of bleeding; peritoneal damage; and mucosal damage. Many teams differ considerably in the type of ancillary treatment afforded the patient: anti-histamines, cortisone, antibiotics, Dextran, hydrotubation, etc.. Very often reports of additional infertility problems are included in some and excluded in others: e.g., anovulation, an history of previous infertility surgery.

The reported term pregnancy rate following salpingo-ovariolysis by conventional techniques vary between 30% and 60% with an ectopic pregnancy rate of 2-5%. Diamond reported a microsurgical result of 57.1% when compared to his earlier group of patients operated by the conventional technique of 25%. A similar report was published by Gomel , but without a comparative study.

Whereas there are many reports of results following microsurgical salpingostomy, involving many additional fertility factors, there are precious few reports following the performance of salpingo-ovariolysis alone. Interestingly, with the advent of increased laparoscopic lysis of adhesions, the reported results are very comparable to those of Diamond and Gomel.

CONCLUSION

As of this date, microsurgical techniques are in wide use. However, many procedures performed by laparotomy using these techniques have been supplanted by operative laparoscopy techniques. Despite ten years of intensive experimental and clinical studies, conclusions regarding effectiveness in preventing adhesions are obscure. The confounding factors are many and patients have been most reluctant to place themselves as possible "controls" where repair for infertility is the major consideration of the surgery. The techniques are changing and the studies continuing, as evidenced by the material within this publication.

BIBLIOGRAPHY

Adhesive Study Group. Reduction of postoperative pelvic adhesions with intraperitoneal 32% dextran 70: a prospective, randomized clinical trial. Fertil Steril 40:612-619.1.

Arronet GH et al. A 9 year survey of fallopian tube dysfunction in human infertility: diagnosis and therapy. Fertil Steril 20:903 1969.

Blandau R. Comparative aspects of tubal anatomy & physiology as they relate to reconstructive procedures. J Reprod Med 21:7, 1978.

Bronson RA & Wallach EE. Lysis of periadnexal adhesions for correction of infertility. Fertil Steril 28:613,1977.

Diamond E. Lysis of post-operative pelvic adhesions in infertility. Fertil Steril 31:287, 1979, Obstet Gynecol 52:591-596, 1978.

di Zerega GS & Hodgen GD. Prevention of postoperative tubal adhesions: comparative study of commonly used agents. Am J Obstet Gynecol. 136:173-178, 1980.

Garcia CR.(1968). Surgical reconstruction of the oviduct in the infertile patient. In SJ Behrman, RW Kistner (Eds). "Progress in infertility. Boston: Little, Brown p. 255.

Gomel V.(1983). Microsurgery in female infertility. p 23. Little Brown, Boston.

Grant A. Infertility surgery of the oviduct. Fertil Steril. 22:496-503, 1971.

Horne HW. et al. The prevention of post-operative pelvic adhesions following conservative operative treatment for human fertility: a final 3 year follow-up report. Int J Fertil 18:109-115, 1973.

Liao S et al. Prevention of post-operative intestinal adhesions in primates. Surg Gynecol Obstet. 137:816-818, 1973.

Martius H. Surgical technique in the treatment of sterility in women. Int. J. Surg. 4:70, 1959.

Replogle, RL et al. Prevention of post-operative intestinal adhesions with combined promethazine and dexamethasone therapy. Ann. Surg. 163:580-588, 1966.

Rosenberg SM&Board JA. High molecular weight dextran in human infertility surgery. Am J Obstet Gynecol. 148:380-385, 1984.

Seitz HM et al. Postoperative intraperitoneal adhesions: a double-blind assessment of their prevention in the monkey. Fertil Steril. 24: 935-940, 1973.

Smith DC. In V. Gomel, Recent advances in surgical correction of tubal disease producing infertility. Current Problems Obstet Gynecol (No. 10): 28-9, 1978.

Swolin K. So Fertilitat Operationen, Tiel I and II, Acta Obstet Gynecol Scand. 46:234, 1967.

Swolin K et al. Traumatization of the abdominal serosa. Acta Chir Scand. 140:203-204, 1974.

Wheeless CR. Problems with tubal reconstruction following laparoscopic sterilization using the electrocoagulation and resection technique. Fertil Steril 28:723, 1977.

Winston RML. Microsurgical reanastomosis of the rabbit oviduct and its functional and pathologic sequellae. Br J Obstet Gynaecol 82:513, 1975.

Young PE et al. Reconstructive surgery for infertility at the boston hospital for women. Am J Obstet Gynecol. 108:1092, 1970.

Treatment of Post-Surgical Adhesions, pages 59–65

PREVENTING ADHESIONS— ELECTROSURGERY: ADVANTAGES AND DISADVANTAGES

Richard M. Soderstrom, M.D.
Clinical Professor of Obstetrics and Gynecology
University of Washington Medical School
726 Broadway (305)
Seattle, Washington 98122

Meticulous hemostasis reduces the chance of postoperative adhesions. Because the presence of sutures, including those declared inert, may enhance adhesion formation, lasers and electrosurgery are popular tools used to keep adhesion formation to a minimum. Both laser and electrosurgery work on a similar biological principle -- the cellular fluid is heated until a dehydration occurs (the process of coagulation) or by increasing the density of power (laser) or current (electrosurgery) the cell membrane explodes (as in cutting). Despite the "Starwars" mystique that surround lasers, electrophysics in surgery has more variables than lasers, making the learning curve for the average surgeon and support staff more tedious than with state of art lasers. It is ironic that laser courses, a weekly event, include a thorough review of the physics of lasers, yet it is a rare surgeon who understands the best way to make the electron do his/her bidding. This document is not a denouncement of lasers nor a promoter of electrosurgical instruments. Its purpose is to encourage the gynecologic surgeon to reassess his/her skills with electrosurgery and use either technology with care and comfort to the best benefit of the patient.

Basic Electricity

Electrons are particles of energy that when pushed (or passed) through human tissue create heat and sometimes destruction. Voltage is the pressure force required to push electrons. The standard measure of pressure is 1 volt. Thus, if we draw the analogy of electricity to water, an electron would be analogous to a molecule of water and voltage would be analogous to water pressure.

Whereas volume of water must be measured in cubic centimeters, the volume of electrons is measured in amperes. Moreover, if we push a volume of water through a conduit at a given pressure over a specific period, we create current. When used in electricity, current means the passage of a given quanity of electrons (ampere) at a given pressure (volts) over a given period. For either water or electricity, as resistance increases, the flow of current decreases. The difficulty of pushing the electrons through tissue or other material can be defined as resistance measured in ohms.

As a last definition, electrical power (watts) is the energy produced or consumed over a period of time. The electrical power may be defined as pressure x current, or volts x current, or volts x electrons (ampere) per second.

Fundamentals of Electrosurgery

Manipulating electrons through living tissue with enough force (pressure) to create heat and, if desired, tissue destruction is **electrosurgery. Electrogenerators** are machines that produce an alternating current of electricity at a frequency that will not stimulate muscle activity (500,000 to 3 million cycles per second). Whereas direct current flows in one direction only, alternating current flows to and fro, first increasing to a maximum in one direction and then increasing to a maximum in the other direction. Because a wave of current is formed, variations in the actual physical form of the wave affect the surgical result.

The wave form of alternating current has a negative pole or peak and a positive pole or peak. The measurement from 0 polarity to positive or negative polarity is called the **peak voltage** of the wave form. The measurement from plus peak to negative peak, which is twice peak voltage, is called **peak-to-peak voltage.** A wave form that builds up to a high peak and then rapidly decreases to 0 (modulated or damped) is called a **coagulating** wave form.

A **cutting wave** is an undamped or non-modulated wave form. A pure cutting wave form is generally produced by continuous energy. Because of this continuous flow, the peak voltage need not be as high as with the damped wave form to create the same wattage. When coagulation effect must be enhanced to produce the same amount of power, however, the damped wave form is preferable; bursts of damped wave forms, separated by gaps of time in which no energy is introduced into the circuit, are pushed through the tissue. For an instant, high voltage actually may be present within the electrical circuit. A combination of undamped and damped wave forms is called a blended current.

As electrons, pushed with a given voltage, are concentrated in one specific location, heat within the tissue increases remarkably. This concentration phenomenon is defined as **current density.** The diathermy generator, an example of equipment using this principle, is familiar to most physicians. Here, electrons are passed through the body by applying two large metal conductors or plates on opposite sides of the part to be heated. The electrons are pushed through the plate called the **active electrode.** Electrons are received on the other plate, the **return electrode** or ground plate, after they leave the body. Because current is dispersed over the entire surface area of both plates, the heat thus generated is of low intensity. If either plate is reduced markedly in size, however, current density (and thus heat) is increased accordingly.

Once the electrons enter the body (conductor) they are dispersed through the tissue toward the pathway of least resistance to the return electrode. Thus, a small active electrode can create a burn where the electrons enter the body. Also, the electrons that leave the body through a small return electode can produce another burn.

Because electrons flow through the path of least resistance, they travel through tissue with the least ohms resistance. If tissue resistance is high but the corresponding voltage pressure low, the current may cease to flow or may search out alternate pathways with lower resistance. When the voltage is increased, the electrons have more "push" to find an alternate pathway. Therefore, one should use the lowest possible voltage necessary to accomplish a given job and be sure that the dispersive electrode is in good contact with the patient and broad enough to reduce current density far below the level of tissue destruction (heat). Furthermore, this reduces to a minimum alternate pathways of electron flow. Such alternate pathways could be through a vital structure where the current might be condensed or where it might lead to an alternate return electrode.

Because laparoscopy is remote control surgery, it is important that unexpected movements of the electrode do not occur. By reducing peak voltage, you reduce the chance of electrons jumping or sparking to nearby structures such as the bowel. A 15,000-volt pressure can push electrons more than 1 cm in room air under certain atmospheric conditions. In contrast, a modern low-voltage generator has a maximum peak voltage of 300 to 600 volts.

These considerations have led the FDA to recommend that low-voltage, high-frequency electrogenerators for laparoscopy should produce a maximum of 600 peak voltage or 1200 peak-to-peak voltage, and that the maximum power should be in the range of 100 watts. Isolated ground circuitry systems are desirable, as is a fail-safe sentinel system, should ineffective or incomplete grounding be present.

Biological Behavior of Electrosurgery and CO_2 Lasers

As mentioned, the performance at the end of an electrode depends on the shape of the electrode, the frequency and wave modulation, peak to peak voltage and current and output impedance. The tissue may be cut in a smooth, deliberate fashion without arching, or it can be burned and charred. This great variation of tissue effects is frequently ignored or misunderstood, which is why some surgeons claim that the laser provides better control of the energy needs and provides better wound healing.

Electrocoagulation may be carried out in many different forms -- from slow, delicate contact coagulation, especially with bipolar forceps, to the charring effects of the spray coagulation mode, at times leading to carbonization. The temperature differences may vary between 100 degrees C to over 500 degrees C.

The CO_2 laser beam, with fewer variables, has a cutting effect similar to electrosurgery but can be made to mimic spray coagulation. Because there are fewer variables with the laser, the cut can be more uniform and perhaps with more control and predictability. At times this may be an advantage; at others it may be limiting.

Electrosurgical electrodes can be sculptured to perform certain tasks. A microneedle, a knife, a wire loop or even a scissor can be shaped and sized to a specific duty. When the wave form variable is added, "cutters" can be made to coagulate and "coagulators" can be made to cut. Interwoven into these acts are the output intensity and output impedance characteristics of the different electrogenerators. Finally, the mechanics of a forcep compressing tissue or a scissor cutting tissue will add a dimension the laser cannot do. A laser cannot manipulate tissue as can an active electrode. One electrode that deserves special mention is the suction electrode that can coagulate a "wet"

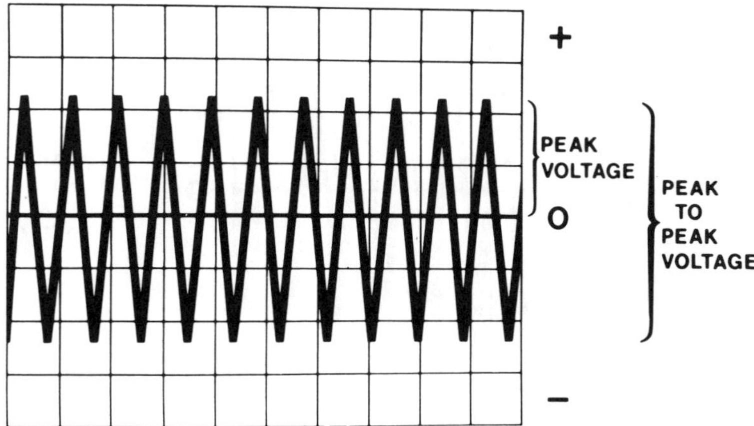

Figure 1. Alternating current generator principle shown with definition of voltage.

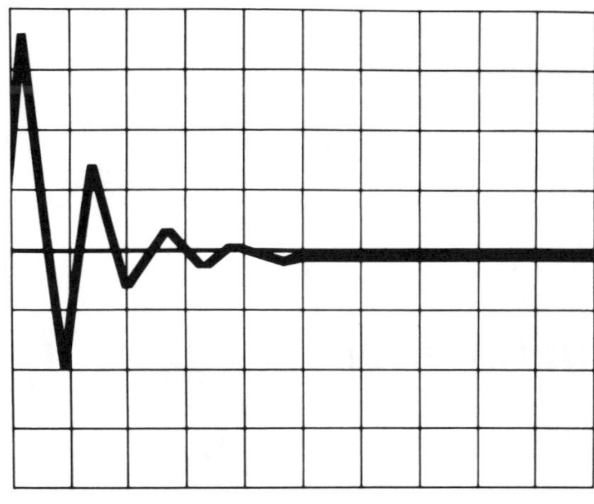

Damped Waves

Figure 2. Alternating current generator with coagulating wave form or spark-gap form.

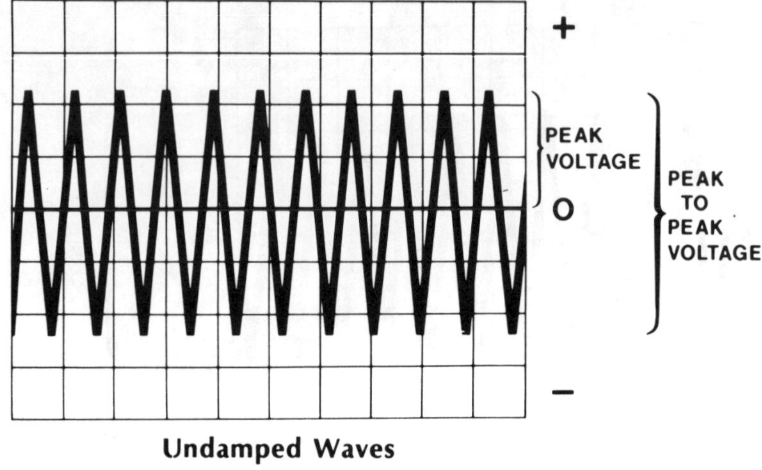

Figure 3. Pure or cutting wave form is illustrated.

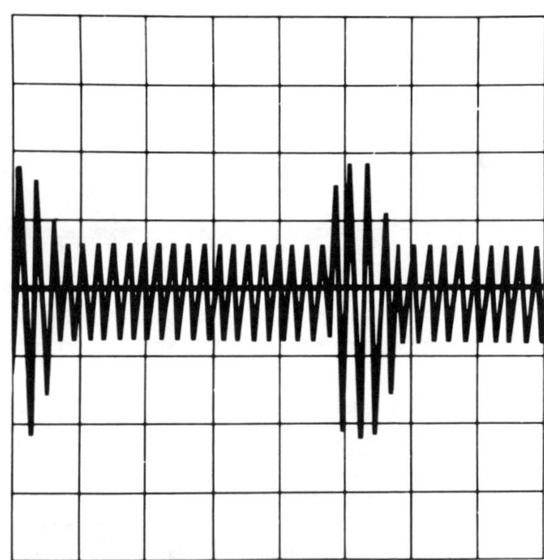

Figure 4. Combined or blended waves give cutting-coagulation effect.

field which would be impervious to the CO_2 laser.

In electrosurgery via endoscopy, the smoke problem encountered with the CO_2 laser is seldom a problem, especially when a non-modulated wave form is used. Finally, a good electrosurgical system, with proper accessory electrodes, is only ten percent of the cost of the average laser.

As we enter the 1990s, the YAG laser is being used with optical fibers and an array of sapphire tips that mimic the different shapes of the "old-fashioned" electrodes of the past. The CO_2 "fiber guide" has been developed to give the surgeon the manual control he/she enjoyed in the "old days" of electrocoagulation via laparoscopy.

A Difference to be a Difference

A difference, to be a difference, must make a difference. In December 1987, Luciano and colleagues studied the immediate and late effects of the CO_2 laser and the microelectrode on the immediate and late effects of depth and extent of injury when the power density of each modality was similar. Their study, in rabbits, failed to show any difference in tissue injury, healing, or later adhesion formation. To date, the clinical studies touting the benefits of laser over electrosurgery have not been convincing.

Summary

Though electrosurgery has been with us for decades, few surgeons have received formal training in its potential uses. The erroneous belief that electrosurgery techniques increase scar formation or impair healing processes, has led surgeons to other methods to deliver energy to the living cell. At the cellular level, a watt, is a watt, is a watt -- knowing how to calculate and administer that energy is the challenge. Laser technology has forced the bio-electrical engineers to develop improved electrogenerators and accessories that are easier to understand and control. The use of digital reader boards, displayed in watts rather than an arbitrary dial setting is one example. A current flow meter for bipolar forceps will now tell the surgeon when all of the tissue has been desiccated.

Soon I hope the power density and wattage delivered at the electrode tip will be easily displayed for the biogynecologic surgeons. Who knows, one day we may have a "laser-electrode" system to meet all of our needs.

Treatment of Post Surgical Adhesions, pages 67–76

LASER SURGERY AND ADHESION FORMATION

William R. Keye, Jr., M.D.
Department of Obstetrics and Gynecology
University of Utah Health Sciences Center
50 North Medical Drive
Salt Lake City, Utah 84132

For the past decade gynecologic laser surgeons have promoted the use of the laser for the treatment of pelvic pathology because of their belief that its use was followed by less bleeding, less tissue trauma, better clinical results, and fewer postoperative adhesions than traditional surgical techniques. However, many skeptics, questioning the validity of these claims, have continued to use traditional microsurgical techniques. Does the use of the laser result in fewer adhesions than the use of standard microsurgical techniques performed without the laser? Can the additional expense and training associated with the laser be justified on the basis of fewer postoperative adhesions? A review of the literature sheds some light on these questions.

ANIMAL STUDIES

In 1983 Fayez and his co-workers compared tubal resection and reconstruction using the CO_2 laser with similar procedures performed with a unipolar micro-electrode on 40 New Zealand white rabbits that they assigned into four groups of ten (Fayez et al., 1983). The animals in the first group had a short segment of fallopian tube resected with micro-scissors followed by anastomosis of the cut ends in a single-layer with 8-0 Vicryl sutures. In the second group, a short segment was resected using a CO_2 laser (1.8 mm spot, 20 W, 900 W/sq cm), and the cut ends were anastomosed in a single layer with 8-0 Vicryl. In the third group a small segment was removed using the laser in a fashion identical to that used in group 2, and the cut ends of the tubes were welded together using the CO_2 laser (no parameters given). In the fourth group short segments of each fallopian tube were resected using a microelectrode (no parameters given) and the cut ends anastomosed with 8-0 Vicryl sutures.

All of the animals whose tubes were resected using the scissors or electrode and sutured conceived. However, only four of ten whose tubes were resected with the laser and sutured conceived, and none of those whose tubes were welded conceived. From these results they concluded that the CO_2 laser beam used according to the parameters in this study had no place in the resection or anastomoses of fallopian tubes. However, they did not state whether these conclusions referred to humans or to rabbits.

Notably, several features of their study design limited the interpretation of their results. First, they used rabbits whose fallopian tubes are anatomically different from human fallopian tubes. Second, the spot size of the CO_2 laser beam of 1.8 mm is extremely large in comparison to the diameter of the rabbit fallopian tube. Generally, a spot size of 0.50 mm or less is used with the CO_2 laser to section a human fallopian tube, a structure that is many times larger than a rabbit fallopian tube. Third, the tubes were cut using extremely low power densities in a continuous mode. The current technique for sectioning human fallopian tubes utilizes the superpulse mode and peak power densities of several hundred thousand watts per centimeter which limits markedly the volume of tissue damaged by the laser.

In a study comparing the effect of the CO_2 laser and electrocautery or peritoneal healing in the rabbit, Bellina and co-workers concluded that the laser produced fewer adhesions and less tissue injury (Bellina et al., 1984). They made incisions of the peritoneum with either a CO_2 laser (12,500 W/cm^2) or an electrosurgical needle and assessed adhesion formation and tissue damage at 0, 5, 10, 15, 20, and 25 days. In all animals treated with an electrosurgical incision, they found adhesions present at all intervals from day 5 to day 25. In contrast, none of the laser incisions demonstrated adhesions, and the zone of thermal injury was only 10% of that created by the electrosurgical needle. While this study was criticized because there was only one animal in each category, six incisions were made in each animal, making the differences statistically significant. The authors believed that the adhesions formed after use of the microsurgical needle occurred because of the random flow of electrons from the point of contact of the electrosurgical needle and the larger volume of tissue damage. In contrast, they pointed out that the laser vaporizes tissue without contact and in a more predictable fashion.

In a study similar to that of Fayez, et al., Baggish and ElBakry compared post-injury adhesion formation and thermal damage produced by either continuous-wave or superpulsed CO_2 laser beams (Baggish et al., 1986). Using 43 rats, they evaluated both acute and chronic effects on partially or completely incised uterine horns by means of scanning electron microscopy and light microscopy to measure the volume of thermal damage. With these sophisticated techniques, they determined that the amount of thermal necrosis with the superpulsed beam (average power 11 to 27 watts, spot size of 0.2 to 0.44 mm diameter) was from 2 1/2 to 4 1/2 times less than with the continuous wave (10 to 50 watts, 0.2 to 0.45 mm diameter). Their findings demonstrated the advantages of the superpulsed mode when incising or excising tissue. In contrast to the findings of Bellina, they found adhesions in every uterine horn regardless of the mode used, although there were 50% more adhesions following use of the continuous mode than following the use of the superpulsed mode. In addition, the adhesions following continuous mode were denser and more often vascularized than those following transection with the superpulsed mode. Finally, there was less fibrosis following superpulse than continuous mode transections. They accounted for their results by noting that they used high mean power densities between 4,000 and 45,000 W/cm^2 and, in the case of superpulse, peak instantaneous power densities between 100,000 and 450,000 W/cm^2. In addition, the superpulsed mode allowed for cooling of the tissue between pulses, thus limiting the volume of tissue sustaining thermal damage. They determined that the least amount of thermal damage occurred when pulses were delivered at rates of 300 to 500 pulses per second with pulse widths between 0.3 and 0.5 micro-seconds. At higher repetition rates the superpulsed mode mimicked the continuous wave mode. In this study the superpulsed mode created less thermal damage; less inflammatory response; faster healing; and fewer, less dense, less vascular adhesions than the continuous wave mode, even at higher power densities.

In a related study, this same group of investigators compared superpulse with continuous mode on tissue healing and fertility using the transected and anastomosed rat uterine horn (Badaway et al., 1987). They incised the uterine horn with either a continuous wave CO_2 laser beam (20 W, spot size of 0.2 mm) or a superpulse CO_2 laser beam (mean power 14 W, pulse repetition rate of 400, a spot size of 0.2 mm). The subsequent fertility rates were 66.6% in the continuous wave group and 81.25% in the superpulsed group. Significant histologic differences with fibrosis of the muscularis and subserosal layers were found in the group treated with the continuous wave laser beam, but no fibrosis was found in the pulsed laser group. Because adhesions were minimal in both groups, no difference was found in the postoperative adhesion score. These results demonstrated that studies comparing cold knife incisions with CO_2 laser incisions should utilize only high power density, pulsed, laser energy.

In a series of studies Filmar and his colleagues in Vancouver evaluated the CO_2 laser with electromicrosurgery or with surgical microscissors for adhesiolysis and tissue transection. In their first study they created intraperitoneal adhesions in 44 female white rats (Filmar et al., 1986). Two weeks later they evaluated and divided the adhesions with either the CO_2 laser (0.2 mm spot size, 9,550 W/cm^2 continuous wave for 0.2 seconds) or a microelectrocautery needle (0.1 mm tip diameter). Two weeks later the sites of adhesiolysis were assessed. Both treatment groups showed a significant and similar degree of reduction in the extent of adhesions. This led them to conclude that both the CO_2 laser and the microelectrocautery tip were equally effective in adhesiolysis.

In their second study Filmar, et al., compared wound healing after transection of the rat uterus in 20 animals using either the CO_2 laser (0.2 mm spot size; 3,180, 6,370 or 9,550 W/cm^2 continuous mode) or a microcautery needle (power densities of 160,000, 270,000, or 450,000 W/cm^2) (Filmar et al., 1989a). They evaluated and compared scar width, amount of debris, inflammatory infiltrate, edema, exudate, and collagen on days 0, 4, 7, 14, and 21 after the surgical resection. They found that the amount of collagen in the scars and the width of the scars were similar and that the foreign body inflammatory reaction and amount of debris were more pronounced and prolonged in the electromicrosurgery group. They concluded that the more extensive and prolonged foreign body reaction was likely the result of significantly greater amounts of particulate carbon following electromicrosurgery.

In a subsequent study they compared transection of the rat uterine horn with the CO^2 laser and the surgical microscissors (Filmar et al., 1989b). They incised the uterine horn of 15 female rats using either a CO_2 laser (0.2 mm spot, 2 watts, 6,370 W/cm^2 continuous mode) or microscissors. Then the incisions were opposed with 10-0 nylon sutures. The animals were then sacrificed and the wounds examined at 0, 4, 10, 14, and 21 days with three animals in each group. In the initial phase of healing, they noted that the scar width was wider and that the amount of necrotic debris and foreign body reaction was greater in the incisions made with the CO_2 laser than in the incisions made with the scissors. However, by 21 days the wounds were similar. Because of the small number of animals, they did not compare postoperative adhesions. With the exception of an initial foreign body reaction in the wounds made with the CO_2 laser, they concluded that the long-term healing appeared to be similar in the two modalities. Despite these observations they stated that sharp dissection with the scissors is the modality of choice.

Luciano and his colleagues also compared the formation of postoperative adhesions following use of the CO_2 laser and electromicrosurgery (Luciano et al., 1987). Using either electrocautery (tip diameter of 0.15 mm, 20 watts, 88,888 W/cm^2 power density) or the CO_2 laser (0.18 mm spot size, 15 watts, 58,946 W/cm^2 continuous mode), they performed either an ovarian wedge resection or a segmental resection of a portion of the uterine horn. They found no differences in the depth of thermal damage, extent of collagen deposition, or postoperative adhesion formation between the CO_2 laser and electrocautery. They concluded that the CO_2 laser and microelectrocautery are equally injurious to tissues of the rabbit reproductive tract, with no apparent surgical advantage of one over the other.

In this series of animal studies it appears that the superpulsed CO_2 laser was superior to microelectrocautery and similar to the scissors with respect to adhesion formation. However, the implications of these results for humans is uncertain.

UNCONTROLLED HUMAN STUDIES

In the early 1980's the first reports of laser surgery for intraperitoneal pelvic pathology justified the use of the laser on the basis of the assumption that use of the laser reduced tissue handling, decreased bleeding, shortened operating time, and reduced injury to adjacent tissue. Until recently, claims that fewer postoperative adhesions occur with the use of the laser in comparison to more traditional surgical techniques were untested and therefore unsupported by data.

In the first study to investigate postoperative adhesion formation, a multicentered team of gynecologic laser surgeons performed early second-look laparoscopy (<12 weeks' postoperatiivve) in 106 women undergoing laparotomies (Diamond et al., 1984). Using the CO_2 laser (1,000 to 15,000 W/cm^2, 0.8 to 1.0 mm spot size, continuous mode), they lysed adhesions, vaporized endometriosis, resected ovarian tissue or performed neosalpingostomies. In comparing their results with those of another multicentered prospective study utilizing non-laser techniques, they concluded that postoperative adhesions were fewer than preoperative adhesions but demonstrated no significant difference between laser and non-laser techniques with respect to postoperative adhesion formation. Unfortunately, the use of historic controls did not allow the investigators to control variables which may have affected their results.

In a more recent uncontrolled study of 124 women by Donnez, use of the CO_2 laser for endometriotic implants or adnexal adhesiolysis revealed excellent pregnancy rates (>50%) and suggested that postoperative adhesion formation was minimal (Donnez, 1987). Because of the absence of a control or comparison group, he could not conclude that the use of the laser was more efficient than scissors or microelectrocautery. However, in eight patients no pelvic adhesions were found following treatment with vaporization of endometriotic implants.

In a third uncontrolled multicentered study, Daniell and colleagues reported a tubal patency rate of 92% and a postoperative pregnancy rate of 21% following the use of the CO_2 laser for terminal neosalpingostomy (Daniell et al., 1986). Using historic controls, they concluded that the postoperative pregnancy rates were similar between laser and non-laser techniques. Unfortunately, uncontrolled studies provide little data concerning the relative formation of adhesions following laser surgery.

CONTROLLED HUMAN STUDIES

The first randomized study comparing laser and electromicrosurgery for the lysis of peri-ovarian and peri-tubal adhesions was reported by Tulandi in 1986 (Tulandi, 1986). He randomized 63 women with adnexal adhesions as the sole cause of their infertility into either a CO_2 laser-treated group (n = 30) or microelectrocautery-treated group (n = 33). All procedures were performed at laparotomy. The laser was used at power densities of 2,000 to 10,000 W/cm^2; no power settings were reported for microelectrocautery. While the pregnancy rates were the same (53.3% for the laser versus 51.5% for the non-laser), the mean interval of time to achieve pregnancy was slightly shorter following laser treatment (9.9 ± 2.0 months) than microelectrocautery (13.1 ± 2.0 months). Unfortunately, because second-look laparoscopies were not performed, no conclusions could be drawn regarding postoperative adhesion formation.

In a similar study Tulandi evaluated postoperative adhesion formation and tubal patency following neosalpingostomy with either the CO_2 laser (power density of 10,000 W/cm^2) or microelectrocautery (Tulandi, 1987). Thirty-nine women with hydrosalpinges were treated at laparotomy and a late second-look laparoscopy was performed (mean 10.7 ± 2.4 and 9.2 ± 2.0 months). He found that with both modalities the degree of adnexal adhesions was reduced following surgery. Comparing the two modalities, no significant differences were found in postoperative adhesions, in the rate of re-occlusion of the hydrosalpinx, or in the rate of fimbrial phimosis.

Finally, Barbot and his colleagues compared adhesiolysis with the CO_2 laser (power density of 2550 W/cm^2) (n = 158) with microelectrocautery (n = 136) at laparotomy (Barbot, 1987). At the time of early second-look laparoscopy (eight days postoperatively) no statistically significant difference in postoperative adhesion formation was found between the two groups. Unfortunately, the patients were not randomized into the two groups, thus limiting the strength of the conclusions drawn by the authors.

CONCLUSIONS

The studies reviewed in this paper are important steps in establishing the relative value of the laser in reproductive surgery and in the prevention of postoperative adhesions. Unfortunately, the animal studies, while controlled, suffered from small numbers of observations; inappropriate parameters of spot size, power densities, or pulse characteristics; and inappropriate animal models. As a result, the implications of these studies for the patient and her surgeon are severely limited.

The uncontrolled human studies substantiate the fact that skillful reproductive surgeons can achieve acceptable clinical results with the CO_2 laser. However, the use of historic controls does not make it possible to discount the possible role of patient selection, presence or absence of other causes of infertility, use of adjuvant therapies, or skill of the surgeon. Clearly, we cannot conclude from these uncontrolled studies whether or not the use of the laser is followed by better clinical results or by fewer postoperative adhesions than with the more traditional non-laser techniques.

Finally, the controlled studies of Tulandi and Barbot and colleagues should be recognized for their unique contribution to our discipline. These pioneers have accomplished something that for other surgeons is difficult, if not impossible, to achieve; that is, to set aside personal biases and the biases of patients in order to randomize surgical treatments. Fueled by the favorable publicity on lasers, surgeons now encounter patients who demand laser surgery. Too often, they yield to patient wishes when, in fact, equivalent results could be achieved using non-laser technologies that cost less.

Unfortunately, even controlled studies do not address the real clinical questions posed by each reproductive surgeon, "For this patient and in my hands is the laser the most appropriate instrument to perform this procedure? Will the clinical results be superior and the development of postoperative adhesions less if I use the laser?" Answers to these questions can be determined only by each individual surgeon who considers his mix of patients, the conditions of his operating room, his skills, and the circumstances under which he generally operates. Importantly, the controlled studies by research-oriented reproductive surgeons in large teaching centers cannot always be translated into the experience of the full-time clinician who performs surgery in a local community hospital. Differences in training, manual dexterity, quality of instruments, assistance and support cannot be factored into the tightly controlled studies of the "experts." I believe that each surgeon must begin to evaluate his own results and determine whether the laser, in his hands and for his patients, is superior to non-laser techniques.

BIBLIOGRAPHY

Fayez JA, McComb JS, Harper MA (1983). Comparison of tubal surgery with the CO_2 laser and the unipolar microelectrode. Fertil Steril 40:476.

Bellina JH, Hemmings R, Voros JE, Ross LF (1984). Carbon dioxide laser and electrosurgical wound study with an animal model: A comparison of tissue damage and healing patterns in peritoneal tissue. Am J Obstet Gynecol 148:327.

Baggish MS, ElBakry MM (1986). Comparison of electronically superpulsed and continous-wave CO_2 laser on the rat uterus horn. Fertil Steril 45:120.

Badawy SZA, ElBakry MM, Baggish MS (1987). Comparative study of continuous and pulsed CO_2 laser on tissue healing and fertility outcome in tubal anastomosis. Fertil Steril 47:843.

Filmar S, Gomel V, McComb P (1986). The effectiveness of CO_2 laser and electromicrosurgery in adhesiolysis: A comparative study. Fertil Steril 45:407.

Filmar S, Jetha N, McComb P, Gomel V (1989). A comparative histologic study on the healing process after tissue transection. I. Carbon dioxide laser and electromicrosurgery. Am J Obstet Gynecol 160:1062.

Filmar S, Jetha N, McComb P, Gomel V (1989). A comparative histologic study on the healing process after tissue transection. II. Carbon dioxide laser and surgical microscissors. Am J Obstet Gynecol 160:1068.

Luciano AA, Whitman G, Maier DB, Randolph J, Maenza R (1987). A comparison of thermal injury, healing patterns, and postoperative adhesion formation following CO_2 laser and electromicrosurgery. Fertil Steril 48:1025.

Diamond MP, Daniell JF, Martin DC, Feste J, Vaughn WK, McLaughlin DS (1984). Tubal patency and pelvic adhesions at early second-look laparoscopy following intraabdominal use of the carbon dioxide laser: initial report of the intraabdominal laser study group. Fertil Steril 42:7171.

Donnez J (1987). CO_2 laser laparoscopy in infertile women with endometriosis and women with adnexal adhesions. Fertil Steril 48:390.

Daniell JF, Diamond MP, McLaughlin DS, Martin DC, Feste J, Surrey MW, Friedman S, Vaughn WK (1986). Clinical results of terminal salpingostomy with the use of the CO_2 laser: Report of the intraabdominal laser study group. Fertil Steril 45:175.

Tulandi T (1986). Salpingo-ovariolysis: a comparison between laser surgery and electrosurgery. Fertil Steril 45:489.

Tulandi T (1987). Adhesion formation after reproductive surgery with and without the carbon dioxide laser. Fertil Steril 47:704.

Barbot J, Parent B, Dubuisson JB, Aubriot FX (1987). A clinical study of the CO_2 laser and electrosurgery for adhesiolysis in 172 cases followed by early second-look laparoscopy. Fertil Steril 48:140.

Treatment of Post Surgical Adhesions, pages 77–83

EARLY SECOND LOOK LAPAROSCOPY

Trudy C.M. Trimbos-Kemper, J. Baptist Trimbos, Eylard V. van Hall

Department of Gynecology and Reproduction, Leiden University Medical Centre, The Netherlands.

INTRODUCTION

We have started to perform early second look laparoscopy (ESLL) following tubal surgery in our department since 1980. The objective of the procedure was to prevent adhesion formation after adhesiolysis, fimbriolysis and salpingostomy and to enhance the fertility prognosis of patients suffering from tubal infertility.

ESLL was performed on the eighth postoperative day. It has been shown that postoperative adhesions begin to form on the third post-operative day and that formation is mostly complete by 21 days. (Johnson and Whitting, 1962; Ellis, 1980)
After eight days the adhesions are still gelatinous and soft and without vascular infiltration allowing for easy removal and general lack of significant bleeding. Furthermore, it proved to be a practical and psychological advantage to perform ESLL during the same hospital admission of tubal surgery.

OPERATIVE TECHNIQUE

ESLL is performed under general anesthesia. The double puncture technique is used, requiring some caution so as not to provoke dehiscence of the fresh Pfannenstiel wound. Therefore, the second puncture should be made at least 4 cm cephalad of this wound. The internal genitals are then thoroughly inspected and adhesions, if any, loosened up by moving the laparoscopic probe along them. If any bleeding is provoked the small pelvis is rinsed with saline. Tubal patency is checked again by hydrotubation with methylene blue and the abdominal cavity is instilled with 100 ml 32% dextran 70. On average the procedure takes no more than 15 minutes. Patient acceptation of ESLL is generally good (10 refusals in 500 consecutive cases). The day after ESLL the patient is discharged.

COMPLICATIONS

Bleeding from the second puncture side, necessitating laparotomy to stop the hemorrhage occurred once in 500 ESLL's (2‰). Less severe bleeding form the second look laparoscopic puncture was seen in six out of 500 ESLL's (12‰). In all these cases bleeding could be controlled by pressure or a deep ligature in the anterior abdominal wall. A small dehiscence of the Pfannenstiel wound was provoked in two patients in the early years of ESLL. After we had moved the second puncture site a couple of centimeters more cephalad, this problem was not encountered again.

Leakage of 32% dextran 70 from the laparoscopic second puncture occurred in 15 out of 500 cases (3%). In all cases the leakage stopped spontaneously. In one of these 15 cases dextran leakage entered into the subcutaneous space as far as the vulvar area. Total resorption took two weeks in this patient.

CHARACTERISTICS OF POSTOPERATIVE ADHESION FORMATION

The first 188 ESLL's were performed between August 1980 and January 1984. In these cases a detailed analysis was undertaken of the incidence and preferred localization of postoperative adhesions. Furthermore, the adhesions found at ESLL were related to the severity of adhesions treated by tubal surgery and the efficacy of adhesion removal at ESLL was assessed on the basis of a later laparoscopy one to two years following ESLL. In 104 of these 188

patients (55%) adhesions were found at ESLL around both adnexa or the only remaining adnex.
In 39 patients adhesions were found surrounding one of two adnexa and in 45 patients (25%) no adhesions were found at all. The most frequent site of the adhesions was between the ampulla of the tube and the ovary or between the ovary and the lateral pelvic wall or broad ligament. These adhesions were usually easy to separate with the laparascopic probe. In some cases adhesions were encountered between the left tube or ovary and the sigmoid. Such adhesions were often difficult to remove and tended to be tight and more vascularized.

There appears to be a distinct relation between the adhesions found at tubal surgery and the adhesions found at ESLL. In patients with no adhesions at tubal surgery or only slight ones no adhesions had formed as far as could be determined by ESLL in 52% of cases. When moderate or severe adhesions had been treated at the time of fertility surgery, adhesions were present again at ESLL in 70% of cases. This difference is statisticallly significant ($X^2 = 10.06$; $p < 0.01$) (TABLE 1).

TABLE 1. relation between the degree of adhesions at tubal surgery and at ESLL in 188 patients (298 adnexa)

ADHESIONS AT TUBAL SURGERY	ADHESIONS AT ESLL		
	NOT PRESENT	PRESENT	TOTAL
none/grade I adhesions	32 (52%)	30 (48%)	62 (100%)
adhesions grade II/III*	71 (30%)	165 (70%)	236 (100%)
TOTAL	103 (35%)	195 (65%)	298 (100%)

*$X^2 = 10.06$; $p<0.01$

In 64 of the 188 patients a late laparoscopy (LL) was performed 1-2 years after ESLL. This was a selected group of patients because persisting infertility after tubal surgery was the major indication of LL in all 64 patients. In these 64 patients a total of 104 adnexa were analyzed. In women without adhesions at ESLL, LL revealed an unchanged situation in about 80% of cases. In 12% of adnexa analyzed (5 patients) dense adhesions were seen at LL whereas no adhesions were encountered at the time of ESLL. Two of these five patients suffered from intercurrent PID. In one of these five patients intraperitoneal hemorrhage was seen at ESLL that had so far been unnoticed during the postoperative course following tubal surgery. Although the pelvis was thoroughly cleared and rinsed at ESLL, she developed dense adhesions later on.

In 73% of cases the avascular adhesions removed at ESLL did not recur. Of the vascular adhesions removed at ESLL 46% had not recurred at LL. Of the dense adhesions removed with difficulty and bleeding at ESLL, 17% was completly absent at LL.

TABLE 2. presence and classification of adhesions in 64 patients (104 adnexa) at ESLL and LL

ADHESIONS AT ESLL	ADHESIONS AT LATE LAPAROSCOPY*			
	NONE OR GRADE I	GRADE II	GRADE III	TOTAL
NONE	33 (79%)	4 (9%)	5 (12%)	42 (100%)
AVASCULAR	19 (73%)	3 (12%)	4 (15%)	26 (100%)
VASCULAR	11 (46%)	4 (17%)	9 (37%)	24 (100%)
DENSE	2 (17%)	2 (17%)	8 (66%)	12 (100%)
TOTAL	65 (62.5%)	13 (12.5%)	26 (25%)	104 (100%)

*Miami classification

CONTROL GROUP

One of the conclusions of the findings presented sofar would be that ESLL seems to diminish the presence of permanent peritubal or periovarian adhesions. It might be argued however that part of the adhesions present at ESLL but absent at LL would have resolved spontaneously without laparoscopic intervention. This could be verified by performing ESLL as a sham-operation without any manipulation, followed by LL one to two years later in patients who did not become pregnant. Such a study design would not be feasible. Among other reasons it would be impossible to perform an adequate visualization of adhesions without lifting the adnexa with a laparoscopic probe. By this procedure alone adhesions may be removed, therewith changing the laparoscopy into a real ESLL with possible therapeutic consequences. In order to get as close to it as possible we introduced a historical control group of women who had undergone tubal surgery just before the introduction of ESLL. These patients were operated on for the same indications, under the same conditions and by the same three surgeons. The control group consisted of 101 women and did not differ significantly from the study group of 188 patients with respect to age duration of infertility and distribution into the three types of operations studied: salpingostomy, adhesiolysis and fimbriolysis. Nor did we change operating techniques and selection procedures in the five years between January 1979 and January 1984. It was still before IVF became generally available in the Netherlands.

In this control group 69 adnexa could be analyzed by LL. We compared the study group with ESLL with the control group without ESLL with respect to the incidence of permanent adhesions seen at LL. The percentage of adnexa free of adhesions in the control group was 39% as against 63% in the study group. This difference is statistically significant (x^2 9.1; $p < 0.01$). So it seems from these findings that a significant spontaneous resorption of adhesions without ESLL does not occur making a beneficial effect of ESLL in diminishing permanent adhesions following tubal surgery very likely.

PREGNANCY RATES FOLLOWING ESLL

To study the significance of ESLL with respect to fertility we compared pregnancy rates of the study group (with ESLL) and the control group (without ESLL). Follow-up was closed at the first of April 1988, thus ranging from eight to nine years in the control group and from four to eight years in the study group. To compensate for the difference in follow-up duration the actuarial life table method was used.

No difference was found between the intra uterine pregnancy rates in both groups, amounting to 33% and 34% respectively in both control group and study group after four years.

There was, however, a significant difference between the groups relating to the occurrence of ectopic pregnancies. In the study group the cumulative ectopic pregnancy rate after four years amounted to 11% as against 21% in the control group of patients in whom ESLL has not been performed.

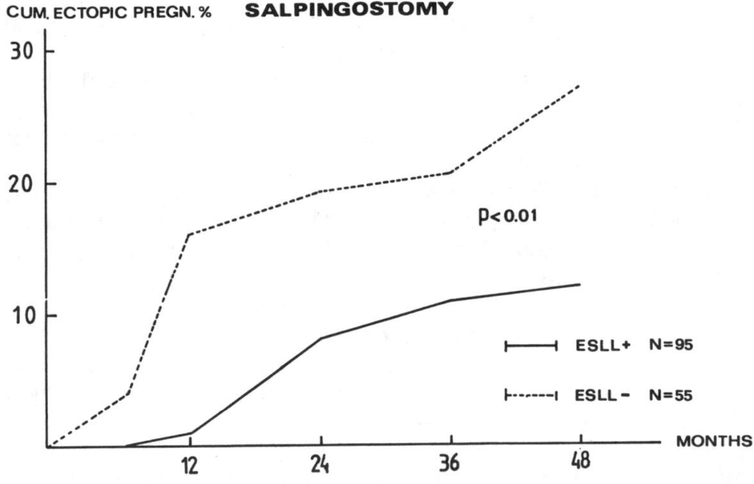

Figure 1. cumulative ectopic pregnancy rate after salpingostomy in patients who did (ESLL +) and did not (ESLL -) undergo early second look laparoscopy.

This different incidence of ectopic pregnancies could be explained entirely through the differences in the salpingostomy group. In patients who underwent salpingostomy followed by ESLL (study group) the cumulative ectopic pregnancy rate after four years amounted to 12% as against 27% after salpingostomy without ESLL (control group; figure 1). This is a statistically significant difference ($p<0.01$).

IN CONCLUSION

Our study has shown that ESLL is a safe and effective method of diminishing postoperative adhesion formation following tubal surgery. Depending on the severity of adhesions removed at ESLL 17% (dense) to 73% (avascular) of them will not recur. ESLL was associated with a significant lower ectopic pregnancy rate after salpingostomy. Intra uterine pregnancy rate was not significantly different after ESLL. The benefit of ESLL for fertility prognosis after tubal surgery other than salpingostomy should, therefore, be critically regarded.

REFERENCES

Ellis H (1980). Internal overhealing: the problem of intraperitoneal adhesions. World J Surg 4:303.

Johnson FR, Whitting HW (1962). Repair of parietal peritoneum. Br J Surg 49:653.

Treatment of Post-Surgical Adhesions, pages 85–91

CLINICAL AND SCIENTIFIC IMPLICATIONS OF SECOND-LOOK LAPAROSCOPY

Togas Tulandi M.D., FRCS(C)

Department of Obstetrics and Gynecology, McGill University, Montreal, Quebec, Canada, H3A 1A1

One of the factors in the failure of a reproductive surgery is postoperative adhesion reformation. Peritubal and periovarian adhesions might impair fertility by interfering with ovum pick-up mechanism and gamete transport. It has been reported that liberation of these adhesions is associated with a better pregnancy rates. One of the technique to remove these adhesions is salpingo-ovariolysis during a second-look laparoscopy.

In spite of the clinical impression that adhesions impair fertility and the pregnancy rates after liberation of periadnexal adhesions is about 50% (Gomel and McComb, 1979; Tulandi, 1986), the value of salpingo-ovariolysis has not been properly studied. Furthermore, Collins et al (1983), reported that the majority of pregnancies among women with "incomplete tubal occlusion" occurred independently of treatment. We recently (Tulandi et al, 1989) evaluated the pregnancy occurrence among women with periadnexal adhesions with or without laparotomy and salpingo-ovariolysis. The cumulative pregnancy rate at 24 months follow-up was 45% in the treated group and 16% in the non-treated group. It suggests that although pregnancy might occur in infertile women who have periadnexal adhesions, treatment with salpingo-ovariolysis is associated with a higher pregnancy rate. Therefore, periadnexal adhesion is indeed one of the cause of infertility. However, no difference was found in the ectopic pregnancy rate between the treated and the non-treated group, suggesting that the intrinsic damage to the Fallopian tube plays a more important role in the development of ectopic pregnancy than the adhesions.

With the rapid development of laparoscopic surgery, more and more reproductive procedures are done by laparoscopy. The advantages of this technique over laparotomy are shorter hospital stay, quick recovery and cost savings. The clinical efficacy of salpingo-ovariolysis by laparotomy versus laparoscopy has not been adequately evaluated. Using rabbit model, Luciano et al (1989) studied postoperative adhesions formation and reduction following laser surgery by laparoscopy versus laparotomy. They found that laparotomy is associated with much more postoperative adhesion reformation than laparoscopy. They also found that salpingo-ovariolysis by laparoscopy produces less adhesions reformation than by laparotomy.

SECOND-LOOK LAPAROSCOPY

In 1967, Swolin reported the use of laparoscopy to evaluate the results of certain reproductive operations. Since then, more studies on the use of laparoscopy to evaluate the result of a given reproductive surgery were reported. Laparoscopy is indeed an important tool for a reproductive surgeon. It has been used to evaluate adhesions reformation after a variety of reproductive operations and to evaluate the efficacy of ancillary measures which are used during a reproductive surgery (dextran, adhesion barrier etc.). This diagnostic laparoscopy can also be extended to become a therapeutic operative laparoscopy. Instruments such as laparoscopic scissors, microneedle cautery or laser can be easily used to assist the fertility promoting laparoscopy. Second-look laparoscopy is also invaluable in assessing and treating endometriosis.

Liberation of adhesions during a second-look laparoscopy has been reported by several authors (Table 1). Some investigators claimed that this procedure might increase the pregnancy rate (Surrey and Friedman, 1982) and decrease the occurrence of ectopic pregnancies (Trimbos-Kempers et al, 1985). Others could not demonstrate the improvement in the intrauterine pregnancy rate after this procedure (Gomel and Taylor, 1986;

Table 1: RESULTS OF EARLY AND LATE SECOND-LOOK LAPAROSCOPY (SLL) FOLLOWING REPRODUCTIVE SURGERY

Authors	SLL (# patients)		Study design	Results
	Early	Late		
Swolin (1967)	-	1 year (n: 24)	Cohort	Introduction to the use of SLL.
Raj and Hulka (1982)	1-8 weeks (n:53)	Up to 2 years (n: 7)	Cohort	Optimal time of SLL appears to be 4-8 weeks after a reproductive surgery.
Surrey and Friedman (1982)	6 weeks (n: 31)	6 months (n: 6)	Cohort	Pregnancy rate after early SLL (52%) was higher than after late SLL (16.67%).
Daniell and Pittaway (1983)	4-6 weeks (25)	-	Cohort	Early SLL may improve pregnancy rates.
DeCherney and Mezer (1984)	4-16 weeks (20)	16-19 months (41)	Cohort	60% of early SLL patients had filmy adhesions, 63% of late SLL patients had thicker adhesions.
Trimbos-Kempers et al (1985)	8 days (188)		Historical control	SLL reduces the occurrence of ectopic pregnancy.
Diamond et al (1987)	1-12 weeks (161)		Cohort	Reproductive surgery by laparotomy is frequently complicated by de-novo adhesions formation.
Jansen (1988)	8-21 days (256)	-	Cohort	Early SLL is safe and effective in reducing adhesions formation.
Tulandi et al (1989)	-	1 year (74)	Randomized control	Late SLL does not increase the pregnancy rate or decrease the incidence of ectopic pregnancy.

Tulandi et al, 1989). These studies differ in the interval between the initial reproductive surgery and the laparoscopy (8 days to 2 years) (Table 1).

Trimbos-Kemper et al (1985), in a prospective study and by using a historical control group, reported that early second-look laparoscopy (8 days after salpingostomy) significantly reduces the incidence of ectopic pregnancy. They postulated that this is due to the easier liberation of gelatinous adhesions at 8 days after a reproductive surgery compared to the more difficult salpingo-ovariolysis of thick, vascular and organized adhesions at a later date. Although, the pregnancy rate was similar, the surgery-conception interval in patients who underwent a second-look operative laparoscopy tended to be shorter than patients who did not have this second procedure. On the contrary, Surrey and Friedman (1982) reported that the pregnancy rate after second-look operative laparoscopy at 6 weeks after a reproductive surgery (52%) was much higher than after the same procedure done 6 months later (16.67%). Raj and Hulka (1982), found that the optimal time for a second-look laparoscopy and salpingo-ovariolysis is 4 to 8 weeks after a reproductive surgery. Indeed in a randomized study, Tulandi et al (1989), found that late second-look operative laparoscopy 1 year after a reproductive surgery does not increase the pregnancy rate or decrease the incidence of ectopic pregnancy. Clearly, late second-look laparoscopy 1 year following a reproductive surgery is ineffective. It remains to be seen with an ethical randomized trial whether early second-look laparoscopy is effective in improving the intra-uterine pregnancy rate.

CLINICAL TRIALS AND REPORTING THE RESULTS

Further studies to assess the efficacy of an early second-look laparoscopy is presently required and a randomized clinical trial seems the best method to conduct such study. Clearly, without a comparison group of untreated but closely similar patients, it is impossible to evaluate the findings with any confidence (Tulandi, 1989). Recent classifications of reproductive surgery (The American Fertility Society, 1988) is one attempt to obtain standardization of various reproductive operations. Randomization may not always be medically feasible or ethically acceptable, but it would be equally unethical to undertake new types of treatment without taking steps to test their effectiveness.

The success of a given surgical procedure is reflected in the occurrence of a pregnancy; in most publications this is reported as a pregnancy rate. It is a simple but ineffective and possibly bias way to assess success of fertility trials, which by their very nature have a variable follow-up time. Life table analysis is more appropriate for such studies and provides compensation for patients who have been lost to follow up The obvious advantage of this method over the use of crude pregnancy rates are such that life table analysis must be considered the method of choice.

SUMMARY:

Second-look laparoscopy is an important tool to evaluate the results of a given reproductive surgery or the efficacy of ancillary measures used during surgery. The efficacy of this technique to improve intrauterine pregnancy rates, however is still unclear. Late second-look laparoscopy does not enhance the pregnancy rate but the efficacy of early second-look laparoscopy remains to be seen in an ethical and randomized controlled trial.

REFERENCES

Collins JA, Wrixon W, Janes LB, Wilson EH (1983). Treatment- independent pregnancy among infertile couples. N Engl J Med 309:1201-1206

Daniell JF, Pittaway DE (1983). Short-interval second-look laparoscopy after infertility surgery: A preliminary report. J Reprod Med 28: 281-283

DeCherney AH, Mezer HC (1984). The nature of posttuboplasty pelvic adhesions as determined by early and late laparoscopy. Fertil Steril 41: 643

Diamond MP, Daniell JF, Feste J, Surrey MW, McLaughlin DS, Friedman S, Vaughn WK, Martin DC (1987). Adhesion reformation and de novo adhesion formation after reproductive pelvic surgery. Fertil Steril 47:864-866

Gomel V, McComb P (1979). Microsurgery in Gynecology. In Silber SJ (ed): "Microsurgery", Baltimore: Williams and Wilkins,p 160

Gomel V, Taylor PJ (1986). Surgical Endoscopy. In Gomel V, Taylor PJ, Yuzpe AA, Rioux JE (eds): "Laparoscopy and hysteroscopy in Gynecologic Practice", Chicago, Yearbook Medical Publishers

Jansen RPS (1988). Early laparoscopy after pelvic operations to prevent adhesions: safety and efficacy. Fertil Steril 49:26-31

Luciano AA, Maier DB, Koch EI, Nulsen JC, Whitman GF (1989). A comparative study of postoperative adhesions following laser surgery by laparoscopy versus laparotomy in the rabbit model. Obstet Gynecol 74:220-224

Raj SG, Hulka JF (1982). Second-look laparoscopy in infertility surgery: therapeutic and prognostic value. Fertil Steril 38:325-329

Surrey MW, Friedman S (1982): Second-look laparoscopy after reconstructive pelvic surgery for infertility. J Reprod Med 27:658-660

Swolin K (1967). 50 Fertilitatsoperationen. Acta Obstet Gynecol Scandinav 46:234-267

The American Fertility Society (1988). The American Fertility Society Classifications of adnexal adhesions, distal tubal occlusion, tubal occlusion secondary to tubal ligation, tubal pregnancies, Mullerian anomalies and intrauterine adhesions. Fertil Steril 49:944-955

Trimbos-Kemper TCM, Trimbos JB, Van Hall EV (1985). Adhesion formation after tubal surgery: results of the eighth-day laparoscopy in 188 patients. Fertil Steril 43:395-400

Tulandi T (1986). Salpingo-ovariolysis: a comparison between laser surgery and electrosurgery. Fertil Steril 45:489-491

Tulandi T, Cherry N (1989). Clinical trials in reproductive surgery: randomization and life table analysis. Fertil Steril 52:12-14

Tulandi T, Falcone T, Kafka I (1989). Second-look operative laparoscopy 1 year following reproductive surgery. Fertil Steril (In Press)

Tulandi T, Collins JA, Burrows E, Jarrell JF, McInnes RA, Wrixon W, Simpson C (1989). Treatment-dependent and treatment-independent prenancy among women with periadnexal adhesions. Am J Obstet Gynecol (In Press)

Treatment of Post-Surgical Adhesions, pages 93–102

GORE-TEX SURGICAL MEMBRANE

Stephen P. Boyers, M.D.[1] and David Jansen, Ph.D.[2]
[1]Division of Reproductive Biology and Medicine, Dept. of Ob/Gyn, University of California, Davis, CA 95616; [2]W.L. Gore and Associates, Inc.

INTRODUCTION

In human reproductive surgery both primary and reformed adhesions occur with high frequency (Diamond et al., 1984a, 1984b; Pittaway et al., 1985; Trimbos-Kemper et al., 1985). While simple peritoneal defects heal rapidly without adhesions (Buckman et al., 1976a), ischemic peritoneal injuries often lead to adhesions (Buckman et al., 1976b; Raftery, 1981; Gervin et al., 1973), particularly when injury sites are adjacent. The anatomic relationship between pelvic sidewall and adnexal structures in humans predisposes to adhesion formation because the infundibulopelvic and uteroovarian ligaments suspend the fallopian tube and ovary across the pelvic sidewall. Large peritoneal defects in this area may arise from surgery for endometriosis or from lysis of adhesions caused by pelvic inflammatory disease. These large ischemic defects are particularly difficult to manage. Attempts at primary closure may lead to further ischemia (Ellis, 1962; Ellis et al., 1965), and free grafts of omentum or peritoneum have generally proved ineffective for similar reasons.

Separation of injury sites with artificial membranes has been reported, but the mechanical barrier approach has been hampered by the fact that most synthetic barriers induce a foreign body reaction (reviewed by Holtz, 1984). Polytetrafluoroethylene (PTFE), however, offers a number of advantages. PTFE is widely recognized as being inert, and expanded PTFE has been used extensively (Matsumoto et al., 1973; Fujiwara et al., 1974; Smith et al., 1975;

Gazzaniga et al., 1976), from vascular grafts and cardiovascular patches to suture materials, artificial ligaments, soft-tissue reinforcements and surgical membrane. These products differ primarily in their physical characteristics. Vascular grafts are manufactured with a relatively large pore size to encourage the infiltration of fibrin and the attachment of endothelial cells. On the other hand, Gore-Tex Surgical Membrane (SM) is manufactured in thin sheets (0.1 mm) with an average pore size $\leq$ one micron. This microporous structure discourages cellular penetration and tissue attachment, and Gore-Tex SM has been widely used as a pericardial membrane substitute in cardiovascular surgery (Revuelta et al., 1985). Examined as long as seven years after placement as a pericardial patch, SM induces no foreign body response and minimal adhesion formation to either epicardial or pleural surfaces, greatly facilitating cardiac reoperation. Gore-Tex SM has also been used experimentally to cover peritoneal defects in the rat, and again it proved to be inert and free of adhesions (Ratto et al., 1986).

REDUCTION OF PRIMARY ADHESIONS

We recently reported that Gore-Tex SM significantly reduced the formation of primary adhesions in a rabbit pelvic sidewall-uterine horn peritoneal injury model (Boyers et al., 1988). In that study, 24 sexually mature female New Zealand rabbits weighing between 2200 and 3000 gm served as the surgical model, which is outlined in Figure 1. All rabbits were operated through a midline lower abdominal incision under Rompum-Ketamine anesthesia using sterile technique. Similar 2 cm x 2 cm ischemic peritoneal defects were created on the left and right pelvic sidewalls by sharply excising a patch of peritoneum. To insure ischemic injuries, each defect was systematically cauterized with bipolar microcautery. The distal 2 cm of each uterine horn was abraded with an equal number of scrapes from a scalpel blade, producing punctate bleeding. After both pelvic sidewall and uterine horn lesions were completed, SM was randomly assigned to cover either the left or right sidewall defect. Each animal served as its own control. A square of SM was tailored to completely cover one defect, overlapping its edges by 2 to 4 mm. The patch was held in place at each corner with a single suture of 8-0 Ethilon (Ethicon, Somerville, NJ). The control lesion remained uncovered, but 8-0 Ethilon sutures were placed at the four corners to match the opposite defect. To further encourage adhesion formation and to better mimic the relationship between adnexae and pelvic sidewall in the human, the ipsilateral uterine horn was suspended across the sidewall defect and was held by another 8-0 Ethilon suture placed 3 to 5 mm on either side of the injury site. The abdominal incision was closed by an everting suture of 3-0 Dexon (Davis and Geck, Pearl River, NY) in the musculoperitoneal layer and a continuous 3-0 Dexon cutaneous suture. Postoperatively, all rabbits received penicillin 300,000 units intramuscularly every day for 3 days. No other surgical adjuvants were used.

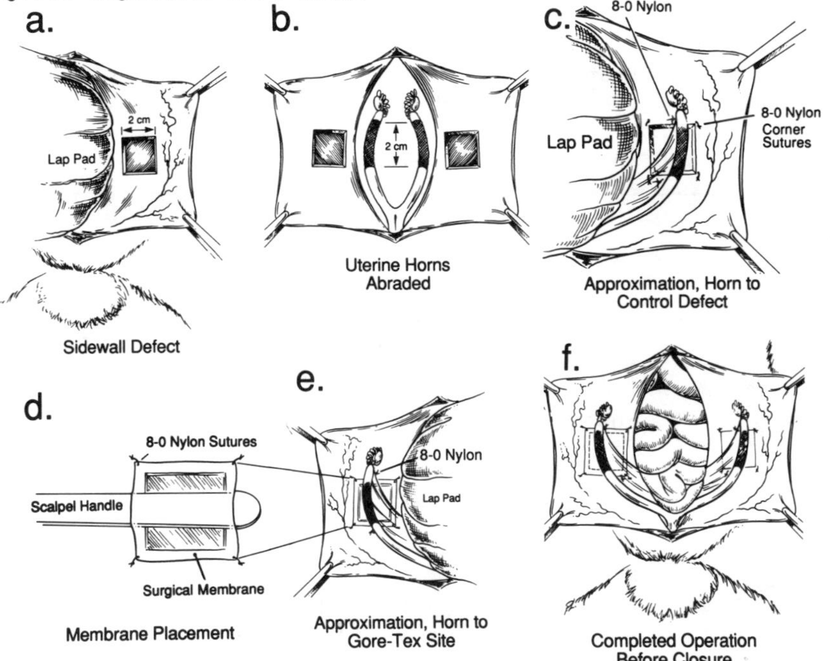

Figure 1. The rabbit pelvic sidewall-uterine horn injury model. From Boyers SP, Diamond MP, DeCherney AH: Reduction of postoperative pelvic adhesions in the rabbit with Gore-Tex surgical membrane. Fertil Steril 49:1066, 1988. Reproduced with permission of the publisher, The American Fertility Society.

Three weeks after initial surgery, all animals were reoperated to assess primary adhesion formation. Adhesions were scored for extent, type, and tenacity, as outlined in Table 1. Total scores could range from 0 to 11. After the adhesions were scored, animals were sacrificed by pentobarbital overdose. Sidewall injury sites and ipsilateral uterine horns were removed en bloc and fixed in 10% neutral buffered formalin for histologic study. Thin sections were stained with hematoxylin and eosin, Milligan's Trichrome, and fibrin stains. Two specimens were also examined by scanning electron microscopy (SEM) after fixation in cold ($4^{\circ}C$) buffered 2.5% gluteraldehyde (0.2 M Sorensen's phosphate buffer, pH 7.0-7.2). Histologic study was performed to give further information about the sites and density of adhesions, the status of the SM-covered sidewall defect, and the degree of inflammation in the vicinity of the Gore-Tex SM. Inflammation was scored as none, mild, moderate or severe according to the number of giant cells, macrophages and leukocytes, and the degree of fibrosis.

Table 1. Criteria for Scoring Adhesions.

	Description	Score
Extent	No sidewall involvement	0
	$\leq$ 25% sidewall involvement	1
	$\leq$ 50% sidewall involvement	2
	$\leq$ 75% sidewall involvement	3
	$\geq$ 75% sidewall involvement	4
Type	None	0
	Filmy, transparent, avascular	1
	Opaque, translucent, avascular	2
	Opaque, capillaries present	3
	Opaque, larger vessels present	4
Tenacity	None	0
	Adhesions essentially fell apart	1
	Adhesions lysed with traction	2
	Adhesions require sharp dissection	3
Maximum total score:		11

Statistical analysis was performed by Chi-square and Wilcoxon Signed Rank Tests. A P value $\leq$ 0.05 was accepted as statistically significant.

Table 2 lists adhesion scores (mean ± standard deviation [SD]) for control and Gore-Tex (SM) covered lesions. The mean scores for extent, type and tenacity of adhesions were each significantly lower for Gore-Tex covered lesions ($P < 0.001$; Wilcoxon Signed Rank Test). The total adhesion score for Gore-Tex covered lesions (4.3 ± 1.8) was also significantly lower than the total score for controls (9.1 ± 2.5) ($P < 0.001$).

Table 2. Adhesion Scores for Extent, Type and Tenacity of Primary Adhesions, and Total Adhesion Score in 24 Rabbits: Control versus Gore-Tex Covered Pelvic Lesions.

	Adhesion Score (mean ± SD)			
	Extent	Type	Tenacity	Total
Control	3.4 ± 1.0	3.0 ± 0.9	2.8 ± 0.7	9.1 ± 2.5
Gore-Tex	1.5 ± 0.7	1.4 ± 0.9	1.4 ± 0.6	4.3 ± 1.8
P	<0.001[a]	<0.001[a]	<0.001[a]	<0.001[a]

[a]Wilcoxon Signed Rank Test

Table 3 outlines, in a two-by-two contingency format, the histologic findings for control and Gore-Tex covered lesions. Light microscopy was used to distinguish true adhesions, either to the uncovered sidewall defect or to SM, from apparent adhesions that were in fact to suture sites. In agreement with adhesions scores, 19 of the 24 control lesions were confirmed to have dense adhesions between the ipsilateral uterine horn and the sidewall defect. In contrast, none of the 24 Gore-Tex covered lesions showed adhesions to the SM itself. Rather, the adhesions on the SM side were to suture sites or to parts of the sidewall defect that had not been effectively protected because the surgical membrane, tacked only at the four corners, buckled between sutures and allowed adhesions access to small uncovered areas of the sidewall lesion. All SM patches remained nonadherent to underlying sidewall by both gross and microscopic assessment. The defect beneath SM was covered by mesothelial cells. The only significant inflammatory response was at the site of the Ethilon corner sutures, where foreign body giant cells were frequently seen. In the two specimens examined by SEM, there was no evidence of cellular penetration or tissue ingrowth.

Table 3. Histologic Findings in 24 Rabbits: Control versus Gore-Tex Covered Pelvic Lesions.

	Histology	
	No Adhesions	Adhesions
Control	5	19
Gore-Tex	24	0
P	<0.001[b]	

[b]Chi-Square Test

Goldberg et al (1987), also using a rabbit model, drew conclusions directly opposite from ours. They reported higher adhesion scores for Gore-Tex covered rabbit uterine lesions and concluded that SM was not an effective barrier for postoperative adhesion prophylaxis. Their study illustrates the importance of surgical design because Gore-Tex and control lesions were not comparable. SM was held in place by multiple sutures, but no sutures were placed around the control defect, compromising their surgical model.

REDUCTION OF REFORMED ADHESIONS

While the prevention of primary adhesions is important, adhesion reformation is probably more relevant to clinical reproductive surgery. Primary adhesions are frequently the consequence of non-surgical injury, as in endometriosis and pelvic inflammatory disease. Lysis of these adhesions is commonly met with recurrence. The definitive study of SM's efficacy against adhesion reformation is incomplete but preliminary data are encouraging.

The adhesion reformation model is a modification of that described above. Bilateral ischemic sidewall defects were induced in eleven mature New Zealand rabbits through a midline abdominal incision, followed by bilateral uterine horn injuries as previously described. We have shown that this model generates dense adhesions between uterine horn and pelvic sidewall at a high rate. Three weeks after initial laparotomy, animals were reoperated through the same incision. Uterine horn-to-sidewall adhesions were scored as described in Table 1. Adhesions were lysed bilaterally using microcautery and microsurgical techniques. After completing adhesiolysis and achieving hemostasis, SM was randomly assigned to cover either the right or left sidewall lesion. A square of SM was tailored to cover the lesion. The SM patch was held in place with corner sutures of 8-0 Ethilon, the opposite side again remaining uncovered as a paired control. Postoperative antibiotics were administered as before. Three weeks later all animals were reexplored and reformed adhesions were scored. En bloc specimens were fixed, stained, and examined histologically.

Table 4 lists initial and final adhesion scores for control and Gore-Tex covered lesions. Initial lesions elicited dense adhesions, comparable to those described previously. There was no significant difference in initial scores for control and Gore-Tex covered defects, but after adhesiolysis, the Gore-Tex side reformed adhesions at a significantly lower rate than the controls. When histology was used to detail adhesion sites, none of the SM covered sides demonstrated adhesions to the membrane itself, but rather to sutures or the perimeter of the patch. The number of animals studied so far is small and these studies are ongoing, but this preliminary data suggests that Gore-Tex may be effective at reducing both reformed and primary adhesions.

Table 4. Adhesion Scores for Initial (Primary) and Final (Reformed) Adhesions in 11 Rabbits: Control versus Gore-Tex Covered Pelvic Lesions.

	Mean Adhesion Score	
	Initial	Final
Control	9.27	9.18
Gore-Tex	9.00	4.73[a]

[a]$P < 0.01$; Wilcoxon Signed Rank Test

HUMAN CLINICAL TRIALS

Gore-Tex Surgical Membrane may have a role as an adjuvant in human reproductive surgery. It's efficacy in humans is just beginning to be investigated. A multicenter national trial of Gore-Tex Surgical Membrane to reduce reformed adhesions between adnexal structures and pelvic sidewall or posterior broad ligament has recently been initiated. Participating centers are Johns Hopkins University, Texas Women's Hospital in Houston, University of California at Davis, University of Southern California, Vanderbilt University, and Yale University. The study is limited to patients with initial adhesion scores greater than 11 by American Fertility Society standards, and calls for second look laparoscopy two-to-six weeks postoperatively to assess adhesion reformation and to remove the SM patch once remesothelialization of the lesion is complete. That study will provide the first information about SM's efficacy in clinical circumstances.

REFERENCES

Boyers SP, Diamond MP, DeCherney AH (1988). Reduction of postoperative pelvic adhesions in the rabbit with Gore-Tex surgical membrane. Fertil Steril 49:1066.

Buckman RF, Buckman PD, Hufnagel HU, Caldwell R (1976a). A physiologic basis for the adhesion-free healing of deperitonealized surfaces. J Surg Res 21:67.

Buckman RF, Woods M, Sargent L, Gervin AS (1976b). A unifying pathogenetic mechanism in the etiology of intraperitoneal adhesions. J Surg Res 20:1.

Diamond MP, Daniell JF, Martin DC, Feste J, Vaughn WK, McLaughlin DS (1984a). Tubal patency and pelvic adhesions at early second-look laparoscopy following intra-abdominal use of the carbon dioxide laser: initial report of the intraabdominal laser study group. Fertil Steril 42: 717.

Diamond MP, Daniell JF, Feste J, McLaughlin DS, Martin DC (1984b). Pelvic adhesions at early second look laparoscopy following carbon dioxide laser surgical procedures. Infertility 7:39.

Ellis H (1962). The aetiology of post-operative abdominal adhesions: an experimental study. Br J Surg 50:10.

Ellis H, Harrison W, Hugh TB (1965). The healing of the peritoneum under normal and pathological conditions. Br J Surg 52:471.

Fujiwara Y, Cohn LH, Adams D, Collins JJ Jr (1974). Use of Gore-Tex grafts for replacement of the superior and inferior venae cavae. J Thorac Cardiovasc Surg 67:774.

Gazzaniga AB, Lamberti JJ, Siewers RD, Sperling DR, Dietrick WR, Arcilla RA, Replogle RL (1976). Arterial prosthesis of microporous expanded polytetrafluoroethylene for construction of aorta-pulmonary shunts. J Thorac Cardiovasc Surg 72:357.

Gervin AS, Puckett CL, Silver D (1973). Serosal hypofibrinolysis: a cause of postoperative adhesions. Am J Surg 125:80.

Goldberg JM, Toledo AA, Mitchell DE (1987). An evaluation

of the Gore-Tex surgical membrane for the prevention of postoperative peritoneal adhesions. Obstet Gynecol 70: 846.

Holtz G (1984). Prevention and management of peritoneal adhesions. Fertil Steril 41:497.

Matsumoto H, Hasegawa T, Fuse K, Yamamoto M, Saigusa M (1973). A new vascular prosthesis for a small caliber artery. Surgery 74:519.

Pittaway DE, Daniell JF, Maxson WS (1985). Ovarian surgery in an infertility patient as an indication for a short-interval second-look laparoscopy: a preliminary study. Fertil Steril 44:611.

Raftery AT (1981). Effect of peritoneal trauma on peritoneal fibrinolytic activity and intraperitoneal adhesion formation. Eur Surg Res 13:397.

Ratto GB, deBarbieri A, Sacco A, Canepa G, Zaccheo D, Motta G (1986). Use of the polytetrafluoroethylene surgical membrane for control of intra-abdominal adhesions. Italian J Surg Sci 16:165.

Revuelta JM, Garcia-Rinaldi R, Val F, Crego R, Duran CMG (1985). Expanded PTFE surgical membrane for pericardial closure. J Thorac Cardiovasc Surg 89:451.

Smith DE, Hammon J. Anane-Sefah J, Richardson RS, Trimble C (1975). Segmental venous replacement: A comparison of biologic and synthetic substitutes. J Thorac Cardiovasc Surg 69:589.

Trimbos-Kemper TCM, Trimbos JB, van Hall EV (1985). Adhesion formation after tubal surgery: results of the eighth-day laparoscopy in 188 patients. Fertil Steril 43:395.

Treatment of Post Surgical Adhesions, pages 103–112

CAN A PRO-COAGULANT SUBSTANCE PREVENT ADHESIONS?

Thomas E. Elkins, M.D.

Department of Obstetrics and Gynecology,
University of Michigan Medical Center,
Ann Arbor, Michigan 48109-0718

The question about the efficacy of procoagulant substances in fostering intraperitoneal adhesion prevention is more complex than is usually recognized. Such substances are commonly employed in gynecologic and general surgery to achieve hemostasis in the pelvis; but have even been implicated, on occasion, in contributing to such problems as dense pelvic fibrosis. Even the earliest description of the adhesion-formation process do not clearly point to the use of a pro-coagulant substance as being important in adhesion prevention. The use of such substances will be presented in the following discussion with an emphasis on the possible mechanism of action that is involved when positive or negative results occur after procoagulant substances are utilized to prevent adhesions.

The role of blood in the formation of intraperitoneal adhesions has been debated for many years. Clinical anecdotes abound in which patients are sighted who have once had a massive hemoperitoneum from a ruptured ectopic pregnancy, who then later conceive in an adhesion-free pelvis. To the contrary, on other occasions the smallest amount of blood associated with the presence of endometriosis or surgical trauma seems to generate dense adhesions in some patients. Earlier literature suggested that meticulous hemostasis was necessary to prevent post-operative adhesion formation, noting the theory that the presence of blood in the intraperitoneal space was a significant factor in the formation of adhesions.(Swolin, 1967 & Gordji, 1975) This was, in fact, one of the earliest reasons given for the success of pelvic microsurgery.(Swolin, 1975) Nisell and Larsson carried out elaborate animal studies using a rat model to determine whether or not the presence of blood, per se, was an important factor in adhesion formation.(Nisell and Larsson, 1978) In observations made from one hundred and twenty rats divided into six groups they concluded that "neither blood nor fibrinogen per se induced adhesions to the serosa of the cecum. On the contrary, a defect in the serosa initiated the formation of adhesions."(Nisell and Larsson, 1978) Their study design used an amount of blood that would correspond to 150 ml of blood in the peritoneal cavity of a woman weighing 60 kg. This study concurred with the findings of Jackson, who noted the completed absorbtion of 100 ml of blood within 48 hours from the peritoneal cavity of dogs in which a Plexiglass window had been inserted into the abdominal wall.(Jackson, 1958) Nisell and Larsson did suggest that blood could possibly enhance adhesion production in an indirect fashion by serving as a culture media for infection, a process known to cause adhesions.(Nisell & Larsson, 1978)

Further, indirect evidence that would question the use of a procoagulant solution specifically to prevent adhesions because of its hemostatic properties come from the controversies surrounding surgical re-peritonealization. Drs. Levinson and Swolin suggested that meticulous peritoneal closure would help reduce pelvic adhesions by covering raw pelvic surface areas after surgery.(Levinson & Swolin, 1980) This would tend to prevent bleeding from the raw surface areas and from the capillary layer of the peritoneal edges around the lesion. However, studies by Ellis in England had demonstrated that reperitonealization could in fact increase adhesion formation, and had suggested avoiding surgical closure of peritoneal edges.(Ellis, 1980) We conducted further studies in rabbits that confirmed the findings of Ellis, and others, implying that meticulous reperitonealization, although it would enhance hemostasis, would increase intraperitoneal adhesions when compared to non-sutured areas of peritoneal injury in the same animal.(McDonald, et al, 1988 & Elkins, et al, 1987)

Of course, the most worrisome questions to confront those determined to use procoagulant substances for adhesion prevention came from the long-recognized usefulness of adjuvant substances with anti-coagulant properties. The prototype agent for many years has been heparin, and it is still used today by many reproductive surgeons in irrigating solutions. As early as 1940, Lehman and Boys presented experimental evidence that heparin could be used safely and effectively to reduce intraperitoneal adhesions.(Lehman, et al, 1940) The mechanism of action of heparin - to inhibit blood clotting and fibrin formation by reducing the formation of a fibrinous exudate over injured surfaces - has been well described as early as 1962, by Knightly and others.(Knightly, et al, 1962)

Into this arena of negative implications for the use of methods or substances that would prevent adhesions by coagulation enhancement came a new set of thoughts about the usefulness of anything that would create a temporary barrier to tissue apposition and thus reduce adhesions. Early studies with heavy molecular weight dextran were very promising.(diZerega, Hodgen, 1980 & Adhesion Study Group, 1983) Dr. diZerega's theories were confirmed by studies done with even more heavy molecular weight solutions, such as carboxymethyl-cellulose.(Elkins, et, 1984; Elkins, et al 1984; Fredericks, et al 1986) The flotation bath effect of these solutions served as a liquid barrier for tissues against adhesions. However, the ideal barrier was still sought...one that would cover surfaces completely and firmly, but only temporarily, so as to allow complete healing of surgical traumatized tissue beneath the barrier without adhesion formation.

One obvious barrier methodology already in use was the number of procoagulant substances applied to tissues routinely for hemostasis. Despite the emphasis on <u>anti-coagulants</u> in adhesion prevention, studies were begun to see if these agents could be helpful "barriers" in adhesion prevention. Numerous studies have appeared now that champion the use of procoagulant substances to prevent adhesions.(Larsson, et al, 1978; Raferty, 1980; Galan et al, 1983; Yemini, et al, 1984; Hixson, 1986) Most noted, with Larsson (1978) that the procoagulant substances being used seemed to form a temporary gelatinous covering over an area of injury. This would serve as a barrier that would separate tissue surfaces while complete healing occurs at a traumatized area. However, in 1984, Lindenberg and Lauritsen, presented animal data showing that a fibrin sealant spray was effective in preventing adhesions in a rat animal model.(Lindenberg & Lauritsen, 1984) Although this sealant contained thrombin, fibrinogen, and aprotinin, thus creating a thin film or gel-like covering over a surface, it was not the type of substance that would provide the barrier effect seen from the liquid "flotation bath" solutions (e.g. 32% dextran-70 and sodium carboxymethylcellulose), or from the solid procoagulant substances (e.g. oxidized cellulose membranes). Therefore, the results of this study raised questions about the mechanism of action of pro-coagulant substances: whether their positive activity against adhesion formation represented a hemostatic effect or a barrier effect.

In an effort to answer these questions, a study was undertaken at the University of Michigan to compare adhesion formation in a rat model between animals in which oxidized cellulose were used, other animals in which a thrombin spray was used, and control animals.(McGaw, et al, 1988) The thrombin spray was selected because it appeared to provide only a procoagulant effect, with a very limited barrier effect being provided (even less than fibrin spray or gel). One hundred and eight rats were used in the study that incorporated cecal abrasion and creation of an adjacent peritoneal defect in order to stimulate adhesion formation. Overall, oxidized cellulose was effective in preventing adhesions, but thrombin spray was not effective. This appeared to verify the use of procoagulant membranes in reducing intraperitoneal adhesion formation, mainly because of its barrier-effect properties, in areas where hemostasis was already achieved.

Further efforts to use procoagulant substances to prevent adhesions have been both rewarding and controversial. The Adhesion Barrier Study Group reported a positive benefit in a large clinical study using Interceed (TC7), a membrane composed of oxidized, regenerated cellulose.(Adhesion Barrier Study Group, 1989) The investigators emphasized the need for hemostasis as well as barrier methodology in adhesion prevention. In fact, it appears that the barrier effect of TC-7 is directly dependent upon meticulous hemostasis in the underlying tissue. However, controversy regarding the effectiveness of procoagulant substances, and barrier methodology in general, persists. Soules, et al, showed a negative effect of most procoagulant substances when compared to 32% dextran 70 in extensive animal studies in rabbits.(Soules, et al, 1982) Soules also noted a difference in the effectiveness of different pro-coagulant substances used as barriers to adhesions. Jansen followed this with an Australian study showing the ineffectiveness of 32% Dextran-70 in reducing adhesions in humans, thus even questioning the "flotation bath" (or "liquid barrier effect").

A general consensus now exists confirming the need to achieve good hemostasis, in preventing post-operative adhesions, especially if a barrier method of prevention using oxidized regenerated cellulose is used. In fact, the use of procoagulants in the face of large bleeding areas promotes adhesions and fibrosis.

But, with the potential usefulness of procoagulant substances becoming more apparent, and with questions about the mechanism of action and the potential for occasional negative effects being unresolved, much potential for future research exists.

At the University of Michigan, work has begun in the re-investigation of the inflammatory response that is the common denominator of all adhesion-forming pathway descriptions. Some newer research is, therefore, focusing on the function of the peritoneal macrophage, that maintains a central role in the inflammatory response. Macrophages are well known for their role in chemotaxis, phagocytosis, and enzyme production. It now appears that they also undergo a "respiratory burst" inducing hexose monophosphate shunt activity, that produces oxygen (-derived) free radicals. These oxygen free radicals (i.e. superoxide anion, hydroxyl radical, hydrogen peroxide radical, hypochlourous acid, etc) have been shown to be tissue toxic in areas of pre-existing tissue injury - thus enhancing and enlarging sites of tissue injury. This has been noted in lung, brain, and gastrointestinal tissue among others.(Fantone & Ward, 1982) It has been studied very little however, in relation to pelvic tissue trauma or injury. In recent years, inhibition of oxygen free radical production has been shown to effectively diminish adhesion formation in a rabbit-endometriosis model.(Portz, et al, In press) Perhaps, even more importantly, substances known to create a flotation bath or a barrier effect (i.e. oxidized cellulose, sodium carboxymethylcellulose, and 32% dextran 70) have been shown not to be responsible for increasing oxygen free radical production, by initiating the "respiratory burst" in macrophages, which many intra-peritoneal foreign body materials are known to do.(Elkins, et al, In press) The stage is set to begin to assess the efficacy of incorporating multiple adjuvants (such as oxygen free radical inhibitors, etc.) with particular aspects of utility in adhesion prevention into procoagulant mediums (such as oxidized cellulose, etc.) or into heavy molecular weight solutions (such as 32% dextran 70 or sodium carboxymethylcellulose, etc.)

In summary, the capacity of certain procoagulant substances both to enhance adequate hemostasis and to provide a temporary barrier to tissue surfaces has made such substances promising additions to the list of helpful adjuncts in adhesion prevention.

REFERENCES

Adhesion Barrier Study Group (1989). Prevention of postsurgical adhesion by Interceed (TC7) an absorbable adhesion barrier: a prospective, randomized multicenter clinical study. Fertil Steril 51:933.

Adhesion Study Group (1983). Reduction of postoperative pelvic adhesions with intraperitoneal 32% dextran 70: A prospective, randomized clinical trial. Fertil Steril 40:612.

diZerega SG, Hodgen DG (1980). Prevention of postoperative tubal adhesions - comparative study of commonly used agents. Am J Obstet Gynecol 136:173.

Elkins TE, Bury RJ, Ritter JL, et al (1984). Adhesion prevention by solutions of carboxymethylcellulose in the rat.-I. Fertil Steril 41:926.

Elkins TE, Ling FW, Ahokas RA, et al (1984). Adhesion prevention by solutions of carboxymethylcellulose in the rat-II. Fertil Steril 41:929.

Elkins TE, Stovall TG, Warren J, et al (1987). A histologic evaluation of peritoneal injury and repair: Implications for adhesion formation. Obstet Gynecol 70:225.

Elkins TE, Warren J, Portz DM, et al (In Press). Oxygen free radicals and pelvic adhesion formation: II. The interaction of oxygen free radicals and adhesion preventing solutions. Int J Fertil.

Ellis H (1980). Internal overhealing: the problem of intraperitoneal adhesions. World J Surg 4:306.

Fantone JC, Ward PA (1982). Role of oxygen-derived free radicals and metabolites in leukocyte-dependent inflammatory reactions. Am J Path 107(3):397.

Fredericks CM, Kotry I, Holtz G, et al (1986). Adhesion prevention in the rabbit with sodium carboxymethyl-cellulose solutions. Am J Obstet Gynecol 155:667.

Galan N, Leader A, Malkinson T, et al (1983). Adhesion prophylaxis in rabbits with Surgicel and two absorbable microsurgical sutures. J Reprod Med 28:662.

Gordji M (1975). Pelvic adhesions and sterility. Acta Eur Fertil 6:279.

Hixson C, Swanson LA, Friedman CI (1986). Oxidized cellulose for preventing adnexal adhesions. J Reprod Med 28:662.

Jackson BB (1958). Observations on intraperitoneal adhesions. Surgery 44:507.

Jansen RP (1985). Failure of intraperitoneal adjuncts to improve the outcome of pelvic operations in young women. Am J Obstet Gynecol 153:363.

Knightly JJ, Agostino D, Cliffton EE (1962). The effect of fibrinolysin and Heparin on the formation of peritoneal adhesions. Surgery 52(1):250-8.

Larsson B, Nisell H, Grandberg I (1978). Surgicell - an absorbable hemostatic material - in prevention of peritoneal adhesion in rats. Acta Chir Scand 144:375.

Lehman EP, Boys F (194). Heparin in the prevention of peritoneal adhesions. Ann Surg 112:969-974.

Levinson CJ, Swolin K (1980). Postoperative adhesions: etiology, prevention, and therapy. Clin Obstet Gynecol 23:212.

Lindenberg S, Lauritsen JG (1984). Prevention of peritoneal adhesion formation by fibrin sealant. Ann Chir Gynaecol 73:11.

McDonald MN, Elkins TE, Wortham GF, et al (1988). Adhesion formation and prevention after peritoneal injury and repair in the rabbit. J Reprod Med 33:436.

McGaw T, Elkins TE, DeLancey JOL, et al (1988). Assessment of intraperitoneal adhesion formation in a rat model: Can a procoagulant substance prevent adhesions? Obstet Gynecol 71:774.

Nisell H, Larsson B (1978). Role of blood and fibrinogen in development of intraperitoneal adhesions in rats. Fertil Steril 30:470.

Portz DM, Elkins TE, White R, et al (In Press). Oxygen Free radicals and pelvic adhesion formation: I. Blocking oxygen free radical toxicity to prevent adhesion formation in an endometriosis model. Int J Fertil.

Raferty A (1980). Absorbable hemostatic materials and intraperitoneal adhesion formation. Br J Surg 67:57.

Soules M, Dennis L, Bosarge A, et al (1982). The prevention of postoperative pelvic adhesions: An animal study comparing barrier methods with dextran 70. Am J Obstet Gynecol 143:829.

Swolin K (1967). 50 fertilitatsoperationen. Acta Obstet Gynecol Scand 46:234.

Swolin K (1975). Electromicrosurgery and salpingostomy: long term result. Am J Obstet Gynecol 121:418.

Yemini M, Meshorer A, Katz, et al (1984). Prevention of reformation of pelvic adhesion by "barrier" methods. Int J Fertil 29:194.

Treatment of Post Surgical Adhesions, pages 113–118

TISSUE-TYPE PLASMINOGEN ACTIVATOR AS AN ADJUVANT FOR POST SURGICAL ADHESIONS

Randall C. Dunn and Veasy C. Buttram, Jr. Dept. of Obstetrics and Gynecology, Baylor College of Medicine, Houston, Texas 77030.

INTRODUCTION

The pathogenesis of post surgical adhesion formation has become better elucidated. The role of depressed fibrinolysis in permanent adhesion formation has been established in experimental situations by different investigators (Ellis 1971; Milligan and Raftery, 1974)). A majority of early fibrinous adhesions are transient and lysed within 72 hours (Jackson, 1958). This is a function of the fibrinolytic system. Those early fibrinous adhesions which remain become infiltrated by proliferating fibroblasts, followed by vascularization and cellular ingrowth, with resultant permanent adhesion formation (Holtz, 1984).

Plasmin is the principal agent of the fibrinolytic system. The inactive proenzyme, plasminogen, is converted to plasmin by plasminogen activators. (Wiman and Collen, 1976) Plasminogen activators can be divided into three major categories: Urokinase-type (u-PA), Tissue-type (t-PA), and other types. u-PA has a low affinity for fibrin such that activation of plasminogen occurs both on surface-bound and liquid-phase plasminogen. This also causes a high degree of fibrinogenolysis (Dano et al., 1985). It is found in several cell types, but is highest in the genitourinary system (Dano et al., 1985). t-PA is several hundredfold times more effective as an activator of the fibrinolytic system in the presence of fibrin than u-PA (Ferres, 1987). t-PA's proteolytic activity is confined to the fibrin surface and has little effect on circulating fibrinogen levels (Ferres, 1987). t-PA is ubiquitous in tissue homogenates which have been studied (Ferres, 1987). Other types of plasminogen activators (i.e. streptokinase, coagulation factors XI, XII, kallikrien, etc.) have high degrees of fibrinogenolysis, immunogenicity, or low specific activation potential for fibrinolysis and have not seemed ideal as adjuvants for post surgical adhesion prevention.

Inactivators of plasmin such as alpha-2 antiplasmin and alpha-2 macroglobulin are ubiquitous and can rapidly inhibit plasmin's activity. However, due to t-PA's ability to bind to the fibrin surface and then induce proteolytic cleavage of plasminogen to plasmin, the plasmin thus formed is protected from inactivation (Matsuo et al., 1981). This sequestration of plasmin after activation by t-PA on the fibrin surface protects it from plasma or peritoneal inactivators allowing for only slow degradation of its fibrinolytic effect. In contrast, free-formed plasmin is rapidly cleared by inactivators (Holtz, 1984; Wiman, 1976).

t-PA is present in both the mesothelium and submesothelial blood vessels of serosal and peritoneal membranes and is responsible for lysing and removing intraperitoneal fibrin deposits (Porter et al., 1969; Buckman, Woods et. al, 1976) Decreased plasminogen activator activity has been postulated to be a possible factor in the development of pelvic adhesions (Buckman, Woods et al., 1976; Buckman, Buckman et al., 1976). When plasminogen activator is reduced by at least 50%, fibrin cannot be cleared and permanent adhesions form (Gervin et al., 1973).

t-PA has recently been made available in pharmacological amounts due to recombinant genetic technology (Pennica et al., 1983). Since fibrin has been suggested to be the pathophysiologic basis of adhesion formation, studies were designed to determine if exogenous rt-PA applied to animal surgical injuries would result in improved fibrinolysis leading to decreased adhesion formation.

EXPERIMENTAL STUDIES

The strongest stimulus to post surgical adhesion formation has been shown to be the presence of ischemic tissue (Ellis, 1962; Ellis, 1982). Therefore, rabbit animal models were established which produced reproducible post surgical adhesions after ischemic injuries were induced. Two animal models were utilized to test the effectiveness of rt-PA. The first was a peritoneal sidewall defect model where 10 square cm. were removed and resutured in place at the corners with silk sutures, creating an ischemic patch of peritoneal tissue. Adhesions uniformly formed in control animals over the entire devascularized peritoneal defect. Scoring system was from 0 to 5 with "4" indicating adhesions to the entire area of the patch and "5" indicating adhesions greater than the area of the patch. Lower scores indicated different degrees of adhesion formation with "0" representing no adhesions observed. In the second model, the pelvic (uterine) model, approximately three cms. of each uterine horn were devascularized by cauterization of their mesenteric vessels and anastomotic branches. In this model, animals scores were on the basis of the percentage of the total surface of the horns which were involved in post surgical adhesion formation. New Zealand white rabbits weighing approximately 2.75 to 3.0 kg were utilized.

Initially, rt-PA was formulated in an inert gel which allowed topical application immediately after the surgical injury was induced and offered potential prolonged effect. This was felt to be useful as depressed fibrinolysis had previously been shown to last for several days (Buckman, Buckman et al., 1976; Raftery, 1981). Results in these two animal models are summarized in Table 1.

TABLE 1. Gel rt-PA as an adjunct to prevent post surgical adhesions. Animals evaluated after 14 days.

Sidewall Model*		Pelvic Model+	
Animals	Score	Animals	Score
Gel Control (n=10)	4.1	Gel Control (n=14)	38.6
Gel rt-PA (0.63 gms) (n=10)	0.2	Gel rt-PA (12 gms) (n=14)	10.7

* Significance at $p < 0.01$
\+ Significance at $p < 0.05$

These results confirmed rt-PA's effectiveness in preventing post surgical adhesions. It also suggested that different total dosages were required with the different models. Though not presented in Table 1, adhesion density scores in these animal groups were also significantly reduced in the gel rt-PA groups.

Additional studies were carried out to determine the effectiveness of rt-PA to prevent adhesion reformation in conjunction with surgical adhesiolysis. In similar rabbits, adhesions were induced by the above mentioned surgical injuries and after two weeks surgical adhesiolysis performed. Topical gel rt-PA was placed prior to closure. Results are presented in Table 2.

TABLE 2. rt-PA as an adjunct to surgical adhesiolysis to prevent adhesion reformation. Animals evaluated after 14 days.

Sidewall Model*		Pelvic Model+	
Animals	Score	Animals	Score
Gel Control (n=6)	5.0	Gel Control (n=13)	51.5
Gel rt-PA (n=6)	0.0	Gel rt-PA (n=14)	25.8

* Significance at $p < 0.01$
\+ Significance at $p < 0.05$

To further determine the efficacy of rt-PA only, without any potential mechanical effect of the gel to affect adhesion formation, it was administered in a liquid form post surgically via an intraperitoneal catheter. Table 3 demonstrates the excellent results when rt-PA was administered. Control and treatment groups had liquid infusions every 12 hours for four days.

TABLE 3. Effectiveness of liquid rt-PA to prevent post surgical adhesions in the pelvic model. Animals evaluated after 10 days.

Animal Groups*	Mean Score	N
Control (normal saline)	35.0	11
Treatment (16 mg rt-PA)	3.75	8

* Significance at $p < 0.01$

Further studies were carried out only in the pelvic model as it was the more discriminating of the two models for evaluating dose response and formulation testing. Excellent results were also demonstrated with liquid rt-PA to prevent adhesion reformation when used as an adjunct to surgical adhesiolysis; see TABLE 4.

TABLE 4. Mean change in adhesion scores after surgical adhesiolysis using rt-PA to prevent adhesion reformation. Animals evaluated after 10 days.

Animal Groups*	Mean Score Change	N
Control (normal saline)	+3	8
Treatment (16 mg rt-PA)	-28	8

* Significance at $p < 0.02$

The results showed that adhesiolysis alone was not effective in reducing adhesion reformation. However, rt-PA was highly successful in reducing adhesion reformation.

CONCLUSIONS

These investigations confirm the importance of the fibrinolytic system as it pertains to post surgical adhesion formation. Maintenance of fibrinolytic activity after surgical injury may lead to the resolution of fibrin and permanent adhesions may not form. Dose dependent results in other rt-PA studies not reported here may reflect that supplemented rt-PA helps the depressed intrinsic plasminogen activator activity post surgically. Dose dependent results which were seen with gel rt-PA demonstrate that it probably acts by a slow release of the fibrinolytic agent (Doody et al., 1989). Since the exact length of time of depressed fibrinolysis after surgery is not known (Raftery, 1981), a single postoperative dose of a fibrinolytic may not be sufficient. Therefore, slow release vehicles, such as the gel vehicle studied here, or multiple postoperative doses may be required.

Possible complications of fibrinolytic therapy such as altered circulating plasminogen activator activity; fibrinogen consumption; intraperitoneal bleeding; or poor wound healing might be expected. rt-PA was measured in rabbit peripheral blood by an enzyme-linked immunosorbent assay (ELISA) with a sensitivity of 3 ng/ml. rt-PA was not detectable with any dose used (Doody et al., 1989). Peripheral blood samples were also assayed for fibrinogen by a thrombin dependent method and no decrease in circulating fibrinogen was seen (Doody et al., 1989). Intraperitoneal bleeding and altered wound healing were evaluated clinically and no differences between control and treatment group animals were identified.

In summary, these data demonstrate that rt-PA is an effective adjunct in preventing initial adhesion formation as well as adhesion reformation after surgical adhesiolysis in animal models.

REFERENCES

Buckman RF, Buckman PD, Hufnagel HW, Gervin AS (1976). A physiologic basis for the adhesion-free healing of deperitonealized surfaces. J Surg Res 21:67-76.

Buckman RF, Woods MC, Sargent L, Gervin AS (1976). A unifying pathogenetic mechanism in the etiology of intraperitoneal adhesions. J Surg Res 20:1-5.

Dano K, Andreasen PA, Grondahl-Hansen J, Kristensen P, Nielsen LS, Skriver L (1985). Plasminogen activators, tissue degradation, and cancer. Adv Can Res 44:139-266.

Doody KJ, Dunn RC, Buttram Jr. VC (1989). Recombinant tissue plasminogen activator reduces adhesion formation in a rabbit uterine horn model. Fertil Steril 51:509-512.

Ellis H (1962). The aetiology of postoperative adhesions. Br J Surg 50:10-16.

Ellis H (1971). The cause and prevention of postoperative intraperitoneal adhesions. Surg Gynecol Obstet 133:497-511.

Ellis H (1982). The causes and prevention of intestinal adhesions. Br J Surg 69:241-243.

Ferres H (1987). Preclinical pharmacological evaluation of anisoylated plasminogen streptokinase activator complex. Drugs 33 (Suppl. 3):33-50.

Gervin AS, Puchett GL, Silver D (1973). Serosal hypofibrinolysis: a cause of postoperative adhesions. Am J Surg 125:80-88.

Holtz G (1984). Prevention and management of peritoneal adhesions. Fertil Steril 41:497-507.

Jackson BB (1958). Observations on intraperitoneal adhesions: an experimental study. Surg 44:507-514.

Milligan DW, Raftery AT (1974). Observations on the pathogenesis of peritoneal adhesions: a light and electron microscopical study. Br J Surg 61:274-280.

Pennica D, Holmes WE, Kohr WJ, Harkins RN, Vehar GA, Ward CA, Bennett WF, Yelverton E, Seeburg PH, Heyneker HL, Goeddel DV, Collen D (1983). Cloning and expression of human tissue-type plasminogen activator cDNA in E. Coli. Nature 301:214-221.

Porter JM, McGregor FH, Mullin DC, Silver D (1969). Fibrinolytic activity of mesothelial surfaces. Surg Forum 20:80-82.

Raftery AT (1981). Effect of peritoneal trauma on peritoneal fibrinolytic activity and intraperi-toneal adhesion formation. An experimental study in the rat. Eur Surg Res 13:397-401.

Matsuo O, Rijken DC, Collen D (1981). Comparison of the relative fibrinogenolytic, fibrinolytic and thrombolytic properties of tissue plasminogen activator and urokinase in vitro. Thrombos Haemostas 45:225-229.

Wiman B, Collen D (1976). Molecular mechanism of physiological fibrinolysis. Nature 272:549-550.

Treatment of Post Surgical Adhesions, pages 119–129

NONSTEROIDAL ANTI-INFLAMMATORY DRUGS (NSAIDs) IN THE TREATMENT OF POSTSURGICAL ADHESION

Kathleen E. Rodgers, Ph.D.
Department of Obstetrics and Gynecology, University of Southern California School of Medicine, 1321 North Mission Road, Los Angeles, CA 90033

Adhesion Formation

Post operative adhesion formation may result from inflammatory responses following trauma to the visceral and parietal peritoneum (Ellis, 1971). Vascular homeostasis is achieved through platelet aggregation and coagulation of serosanginous exudate into fibrinous clots (Movat, 1971). The fibrous bands which are deposited following coagulation may be either absorbed or persist thereby providing a scaffold for the ingrowth and organization of fibroblasts (Buckman, 1976).

Several studies showed that peritoneal macrophage function is modulated by surgical injury. Arachidonic acid metabolites are produced by the PMNs and macrophages present at the site of inflammation or may result from platelet aggregation and may mediate some inflammatory events. Labeled arachidonic acid was incubated with peritoneal exudate cells (PEC) harvested at various postsurgical times and the metabolites formed by the lipoxygenase and cycloxygenase pathways were determined (Shimanuki, et al., 1986). An increase in 15-HETE and di-HETE and a decrease in 5-HETE formation beginning 24 hours after surgical injury was observed. In addition, there was an increase in thromboxane B2 and prostaglandin E_2 (PGE_2) throughout the study interval (2-10 days postoperatively).

These arachidonic acid metabolites may mediate some aspects of the postsurgical inflammatory response. PGs were shown to be involved in events which occur during the generation of inflammation including leukocyte infiltration, edema formation and endothelial cell procoagulant activities (Randall, et al., 1980). NSAIDs inhibit the formation of arachidonic acid metabolites through suppression of cycloxygenase and lipoxygenase pathways and thus lead to a reduction in inflammation mediated by these metabolites (Vane, 1971; Flower, et al., 1972).

NSAIDs in Reduction of Adhesion Formation

Adhesion formation may be enhanced by inflammatory molecules such arachidonic acid metabolites. Therefore, effect of NSAIDs on adhesion formation was examined. NSAIDs were shown to be instrumental in the reduction of peritoneal adhesions. Most studies were conducted using systemic administration of these agents. Siegler (1980) and Bateman (1982) observed a marked reduction in adhesions formation following systemic administration of 7 and 10 mg/kg ibuprofen, respectively, during the perioperative interval. Nishimura found that administration of two doses of ibuprofen after the completion of surgery did not affect adhesion formation (Nishimura, et al., 1984a). However, a significant reduction in adhesion formation was noted after 5 doses (including preoperative dosing) of ibuprofen (70 mg/kg) was administered systemically (Nishimura, et al. 1983; Nishimura et al., 1984b). Oxyphenbutazone, administered perioperatively, in rats and monkeys reduced postoperative adhesion formation (Kapur, et al; 1969, 1972; Larsson, et al., 1977). Further studies were conducted with NSAIDs administered intraperitoneally in an attempt to reduce adhesion formation. Intraperitoneal administration of ibuprofen through a miniosmotic pump, in hydron polymer or in a liposome carrier reduced adhesion formation following abrasion of the parietal peritoneum and serosal surface of the colon (Shimanuki, et al., 1985; Rodgers, et al., 1989a). Tolmetin, another NSAID, reduced adhesion formation after intraperitoneal administration. Very low concentrations of tolmetin, administered in miniosmotic pumps, prevented adhesion formation in the surgical model described above (Rodgers, et al., 1989b). Tolmetin, in a series of micellar (5% Tween 80) and vesicle (multilaminar liposomes) preparations, significantly reduced adhesion formation in a more selective surgical model developed in the rabbit (devascularization and abrasion of both uterine horns) (Rodgers et al., 1989a,b). Most recently, tolmetin reduced adhesion formation when placed in a high molecular weight carrier which may act as a barrier in conjunction with the pharmacologic intervention of tolmetin (Rodgers, et al., 1989c). These data suggest that inhibitors of arachidonic acid metabolism, such as ibuprofen and tolmetin, effectively reduce postoperative adhesion formation.

Mechanism of Action of NSAIDs

There are several possible mechanisms by which NSAIDs could reduce adhesion formation following peritoneal surgery. First, adhesion formation could be reduced through diminished PG synthesis which would reduce inflammatory events mediated by PGs (Randall, et la., 1980). A decrease in leukocyte infiltration and coagulation (which follows platelet aggregation) may decrease the matrix necessary for fibroblast organization. Although PGs are cytostatic agents (Plescia, et al., 1975), and hence a reduction in PG synthesis may increase fibroblast proliferation, without a fibrin, supporting matrix to allow fibroblast organization no adhesion formation would occur. Alternatively, macrophages were shown to secrete plasminogen activator (PA) (Chapman, et al., 1982; Unkeless, et al., 1974; Orita, et al., 1986), which activates the fibrinolytic enzyme, plasmin. If exposure to tolmetin increased the secretion of PA by postsurgical macrophages (evidence suggesting this presented below) then clots would be lysed and no fibrinous bands would form to support fibroblast organization.

A decrease in PA synthesis was shown to coincide with the initiation of inflammation-induced differentiation of macrophages (Bonney and Davies, 1984). Many macrophage functions which are modulated during inflammation may be suppressed in resident macrophages by PG (Bonney and Davies, 1984). Therefore, a decrease in PG synthesis through chemical intervention could allow a more rapid differentiation of resident and infiltrating leukocytes in response to inflammatory signals such as complement and bacterial endotoxin, following surgery. If stimulation of differentiation by NSAIDs occurred, any potential infection present would be cleared more rapidly and would hence be less stimulatory to leukocytes. This, in turn, would allow a more rapid but less prolonged inflammatory response. However, preliminary studies on the effects of tolmetin on postsurgical PEC argue against this possibility (Rodgers, et al., 1988).

Macrophages and PMNs are centrally involved in the initial clearance of bacteria and damaged tissue. Macrophages and PMNs manifest increased capacities including phagocytosis (Ratzan, et al., 1972), superoxide anion (O_2^-) release (Johnston, et al., 1978) tumoricidal/ microbiocidal (Hibbs, et al., 1978) activity following inflammatory and other stimuli which in turn, allow for the rapid clearance of infectious agents. Since many of these functions which are enhanced during inflammation may be regulated by PGs, administration of a compound such as an NSAID, which inhibits PG synthesis (Taylor and Salata, 1976), may modulate these enhanced granulocytic cell functions and alter the kinetics of infection clearance.

Modulation of Macrophage Function by Tolmetin

During peritoneal surgery there are many opportunities for the introduction of bacteria, therefore the effects of these drugs on the microbiocidal functions of peritoneal leukocytes are important. After surgery, administration of tolmetin significantly elevated O_2^- release at days 3 and 5, phagocytic capability at days 7 and 14 and tumoricidal activity at day 3. Differential staining and microscopic analysis revealed increases in PMN numbers at doses of 3 and 10 mg tolmetin (Rodgers, et al., 1988). PGs modulate PMN chemotaxis during inflammation. However, the regulation of homeostasis in the normal peritoneum by PGs is unknown. PG synthesis and release initially decrease during inflammation followed by a concomitant increase in neutral protease secretion by macrophages (Unkeless, et al., 1974; Humes, et al., 1980). Taken together, these findings suggest that PG synthesis by macrophages is necessary to maintain the resident differentiative state of the macrophage. If this is true, inhibition of PG synthesis by NSAIDs may provide the necessary signal(s) to initiate macrophage (and perhaps PMN) differentiation.

Following surgery, there was an increase in the functional activity of PEC (Rodgers, et al., 1988). The phagocytic capability of peritoneal leukocytes was significantly elevated which would allow for a more rapid removal of damaged tissue. By postsurgical day 7, the activities of the PEC from control animals returned to resident cell levels. Administration of tolmetin lengthened the time following surgery during which peritoneal leukocyte function was elevated (Rodgers, et al., 1988). Microscopic examination of PEC indicated that the influx of macrophages into the peritoneum after surgery was delayed by tolmetin administration. In control and treated animals, the infiltration of macrophages into the peritoneum corresponded to the time point at which the early elevations in peritoneal leukocyte phagocytic and respiratory burst activities began to return (Rodgers, et al., 1988). These data suggest two possibilities: (a) PMN activity alone was responsible for the increase in peritoneal cell functions observed; and/or (b) indirect PMN interaction with macrophages was necessary for these elevated functions.

In summary, these studies indicate that intraperitoneal administration of tolmetin elevated leukocyte functions. Therefore, perioperative administration of tolmetin should not increase the risk of infection to the host. These alterations in peritoneal leukocyte function may be the result of a reduction in PG synthesis by tolmetin.

Protease Activity

As stated, NSAIDs may act to reduce adhesion formation through increasing the expression of fibrinolytic activity either through modulation of protease and protease inhibitor secretion or reduction of protease inhibitor activity in wound fluid (Rodgers, et al., 1989d). Therefore, the effects of tolmetin on the levels of protease and proteases inhibitor activity in conditioned media of postsurgical macrophages were examined. Following peritoneal surgery, the level of neutral proteases secreted by peritoneal macrophages increased. Exposure of postsurgical macrophages to tolmetin in vitro suppressed collagenase and elevated elastase activities at early time points after surgery (Table 1). In contrast, the level of PA inhibitory (PAI) activity in cultures of postsurgical macrophages harvested within 48 hours after surgery was reduced by in vitro exposure of postsurgical macrophages to tolmetin (Table 1). These data suggest that NSAIDs modify the ability of postsurgical macrophages to remodel and clear debris from the site of trauma.

Collagenase activity was reduced in macrophage conditioned media up to 48 hours after surgery following exposure to tolmetin (Table 1). These data are consistent with a previous report by Wahl and Lampel (1987) where indomethecin (a PG synthesis inhibitor) decreased the level of collagenase secreted by human monocytes. They proposed that collagenase secretion contains a PG-dependent step (Wahl and Winter, 1984). These suggest that up to 48 hours after surgery peritoneal macrophages was susceptible to modulation by tolmetin (Rodgers, et al., 1989d).

Elastase secretion by postsurgical macrophages was also elevated by in vitro exposure to tolmetin (Table 1). Previous studies by Werb, et al. (1980) showed that purified macrophage elastase could cleave elastin as well as fibronectin, laminin, fibrinogen, proteoglycan, and matrix secreted by rat smooth muscles. Hence, elastase may be important for the clearance of fibrin clots and tissue debris after surgery. The increase in elastase secretion observed after in vitro exposure to tolmetin suggests an additional mechanism by which tolmetin reduces adhesion formation.

A decrease in the level of PAI activity found in postsurgical macrophage conditioned media may result in increased fibrinolytic activity in the peritoneal cavity after surgery. In vitro exposure of peritoneal macrophages, from up to 48 hours after surgery, to tolmetin reduced the amount of PAI activity in macrophage conditioned media (Rodgers, et al., 1989d). Since adhesion formation may be dependent upon fibrin deposition to support fibroblast organization, an increase in fibrinolysis would decrease adhesion formation.

These studies suggest mechanisms by which tolmetin reduces adhesion formation. Tolmetin may reduce the activity of PAI activity at early time points after surgery. Therefore, PA activity may be elevated and in turn plasmin formation would be elevated in the peritoneal cavity. Increased plasmin would then increase fibrinolysis and reduce deposition of fibrin and adhesion forma-

Table 1

Modulation of Protease Activity in Macrophage Conditioned Media by Tolmetin #

Hrs After Surgery	Collagenase	Elastase	PAI
0	71.1±6.3*	272.0±4.5+	45.2±4.3*
6	49.6±9.1*	129.5±1.7+	83.6±2.1*
12	50.7±10.9*	113.5±4.3	65.3±3.6*
24	68.1±4.4*	95.3±6.3	78.4±3.6*
48	60.3±12.7*	101.2±4.0	81.6±2.3*
72	74.5±21.0	99.2±7.5	98.7±10.1
96	141.1±17.2+	94.5±1.4	106.3±4.7

Macrophages were harvested from rabbits at various times after surgery, placed in culture for 4 days with 2 mg/ml tolmetin and the protease or protease inhibitor activity in the supernatant measured

Data are presented as percent of surgical control.

* Significantly ($p \leq 0.05$) suppressed compared to control.

+ Significantly (≤ 0.05) elevated compared to control.

Table 2

Modulation of RBC and WBC Number in Peritoneal Lavage Fluid by Tolmetin in a High Molecular Weight Carrier

	RBC ($x10^8$)		WBC ($x10^6$)	
Hours After Surgery	Control	Treated	Control	Treated
6	205±67	70±20*	67±18	158±76+
12	72±17	42±7	53±9	162±16+
24	77±37	55±11	77±16	95±24
48	31±10	9±2*	31±10	32±5
72	53±10	12±4*	46±9	37±5
96	59±19	12±5*	52±15	26±6*

Peritoneal cells were harvested from rabbits at various times after surgery and the number of RBC and WBC in the lavage fluid was determined. Treatment consisted of 1 mg/ml tolmetin in a high molecular weight carrier.

* Significantly ($p \leq 0.05$) suppressed compared to control.

+ Significantly (≤ 0.05) elevated compared to control.

tion. In addition, acute administration of tolmetin at the end of surgery elevated other macrophage functions such as phagocytosis. This elevated leukocyte function may allow more rapid clearance of tissue debris or fibrin through phagocytosis.

Hemostasis

Further studies showed that tolmetin in a high molecular weight carrier administered in vivo (at concentrations shown to reduce adhesion formation) also modulated the number of red blood cells (RBC) and white blood cells (WBC) in the peritoneal cavity of rabbits following abrasion and devascularization of uterine horns (Abe, et al., 1989). At 6, 48, 72 and 96 hours after surgery, the number of RBC harvested by peritoneal lavage was significantly reduced (Table 2). In contrast, the numbers of RBC and WBC in the peritoneal cavity at 12 and 24 hours after surgery were unchanged and elevated, respectively, in treated rabbits. This reduction in RBC number after surgery could not be repeated with another high molecular weight liquid, dextran 70, or lactated Ringer's solution. These data suggest that tolmetin in a high molecular weight carrier (which may act as a barrier) can reduce bleeding into the peritoneal cavity and thereby reduce the amount of fibrin available to form adhesions.

Conclusion

These data indicate that tolmetin may act to reduce adhesions after abdominal surgery through a reduction in PG synthesis, which in turn reduces inflammation and elevates macrophage functions. In vivo or in vitro exposure to tolmetin modulate the secretion of neutral proteases and PAI activity. The changes that were observed would increase the fibrinolytic potential of the peritoneal cavity, thereby reducing the amount of fibrin available to support the ingrowth of fibroblast and subsequent adhesion formation.

References

Abe H, Rodgers KE, Campeau JD, Girgis W, Ellefson D, diZerega GS (1989). The effect of intraperitoneal administration of sodium tolmetin in a high molecular weight carrier on the postsurgical cell infiltration in vivo. In preparation.

Bateman BG, Nunley WC, Kitchen JD (1982). Prevention of post-operative peritoneal adhesion: an assessment of ibuprofen. Fertil Steril 38:107-115.

Bonney RJ, Davies P (1984). Possible autoregulatory functions of the secretory products of mononuclear phagocytes. Comtemporary Topics in Immunology 10:199-223.

Buckman RF, Buckman PD, Hufnagel HV, Coldwell RA (1976). A physiologic basis for the adhesion-free healing of deperitonealized surfaces. J Surg Res 20:1-5.

Chapman HA, Vavrin Z, Hibbs JB (1982). Macrophage fibrinolytic activity: identification of two path ways of plasmin formation by intact cells and of a plasminogen activator inhibitor. Cell 28:653-662.

Ellis H (1971). The etiology of post operative abdominal adhesion. B J Surg 50:10.

Flower R, Gryglewski R, Herbaczynska-Cedro K, Vane JR (1972). Effects of anti-inflammatory drugs on prostaglandin biosynthesis. Nature New Biol 238:104-106.

Hibbs JB, Chapman HA, Weinberg JB (1978). The macrophage as an antineoplastic surveillance cell: biological perspective. J Reticoloendothel Soc 24:549-556.

Humes JL, Burger G, Galavage M, Keuhl FA, Wightman PD, Dahlgren ME, Davies P, Bonney RJ (1980). The diminished production of arachidonic acid oxygenation products by elicited mouse peritoneal macrophages: possible mechanisms. J Immun 124:2110-2116.

Johnston RB, Godzik CA, Cohn ZA (1978). Increases superoxide anion production by immunologically activated and chemically elicited macrophages. J Exp Med 142:115-122.

Kapur BML, Gulati SM, Talwar JR (1972). Prevention of reformation of peritoneal adhesions: effect of oxyphenbutazone, proteclytic enzymes from carica papaya, and dextrose 40. Arch Surg 105:761-766.

Kapur BML, Talwar JL, Gulati SM (1969). Oxyphenbutazone-anti-inflammatory agent-in prevention of peritoneal adhesions. Arch Surg 98:301-302.

Larsson B, Svanberg SG, Swolin K (1977). Oxybutazone-an adjuvant to be used in the prevention of adhesions in operations for fertility. Fertil Steril 28:807-808.

Movat, H.Z. (1971). The acute inflammatory reaction. In H.Z. Movat (ed): "Inflammation, Immunity and Hypersensitivity," New York: Harper and Row, pp 1.

Nishimura, K., Nakamura, R.M. and diZerega, G.S. (1983). Biochemical evaluation of postsurgical wound repair: prevention of intraperitoneal adhesion formation with ibuprofen. J. Surg. Res. 34:219-226.

Nishimura K, Shimanuki T, diZerega GS (1984a). Ibuprofen in the prevention of experimentally induced postoperative adhesions. Amer J Med 102-106.

Nishimura K, Nakamura RM, diZerega GS (1984b). Ibuprofen inhibition of postsurgical adhesion formation: a time and dose response biochemical evaluation in rabbits. J Surg Res 36:115-124.

Orita H, Gale J, Campeau JD, Nakamura RM, diZerega GS (1986). Differential secretion of plasminogen activator by post-surgical activated macrophages. J Surg Res 41:569-573.

Plescia OJ, Smith AH, Greenwich K (1975). Subverson of Immune system by tumor cells and the role of prostaglandins. PNAS 72:1848-1853.

Randall RW, Eakins KE, Higgs GA (1980). Inhibition of arachidonic acid cyclo-oxygenase and lipo-oxygenase activities by indomethacin and compound BW755. Agents and Actions 10:553-555.

Ratzan KR, Musher DM, Keusch GT, Weinstein L (1972). Correlation of increased metabolic activities resistance to infection, enhanced phagocytosis and inhibition of bacterial growth by macrophages from listeria and BCG-infected mice. Infect Immun 5:499-503.

Rodgers K, Ellefson D, Girgis W, Scott L, diZerega GS (1988). Effects of tolmetin sodium dihydrate on normal and postsurgical peritoneal cell function. Int J Immunopharmac 10:111-120.

Rodgers KE, Bracken K, Richer L, Girgis W, diZerega GS (1989a). Inhibition of postsurgical adhesions by liposomes containing nonsteroidal anti-inflammatory drugs. International Journal of Infertility, in press.

Rodgers K, Girgis W, Johns D, diZerega GS (1989b). Intraperitoneal tolmetin prevents postsurgical adhesion formation in rabbits. International Journal of Infertility. 34: in press.

Rodgers KE, Johns DJ, Girgis W, diZerega GS (1989c). Prevention of adhesion formation after intraperitoneal administration of tolmetin in a high molecular weight carrier. In preparation.

Rodgers KE, Ellefson D, Girgis W, diZerega GS (1989d). Protease and protease inhibitor secretion by postsurgical macrophages following in vitro exposure to tolmetin. Immunopharmacology, In preparation.

Shimanuki T, Nishimura K, diZerega GS (1985). Prevention of postoperative peritoneal adhesions in rabbits with ibuprofen. Sem Reprod Endocrin 3:295-300.

Shimanuki T, Nakamura RM, diZerega GS (1986). A kinetic analysis of peritoneal fluid cytology and arachidonic acid metabolism after abrasion and reabrasion of rabbit peritoneum. J Surg Res 41:245.

Siegler AM, Kontopoulos V, Wang CE (1980). Prevention of post-operative adhesions in rabbits with ibuprofen, a nonsteriodal anti-inflammatory agent. Fertil Steril 34:46-49.

Taylor RJ, Salata JJ (1976). Inhibition of prostaglandin synthetase by tolmetin (Tolectin, McN-2559), a new non-steroidal anti-inflammatory agent. Biochem Pharmac 25:2479-2484.

Unkeless JC, Gordon S, Reich S (1974). Secretion of plasminogen activator by stimulated macrophages. J Exp Med 139:834-850.

Vane JR (1971). Inhibition of prostaglandin synthesis as a mechanism of action for aspirin-like drugs. Nature New Biol 231:232-235.

Wahl LM, Lampel LL (1987). Regulation of human peripherial blood monocyte collagenase by prostaglandins and anti-inflammatory drugs. Cell Immunol 105:411.

Wahl LM, Winter CC (1984). Regulation of guinea pig macrophage collagenase by dexamethasome and colchicine. Arch Biochem Biophys 230:661.

Werb Z, Banda MJ, Jones PA (1980). Degradation of connective tissue by macrophages: I. Proteolysis of elastin, glycoproteins and collagen by proteinases isolated from macrophages. J Exp Med 152:1340.

Treatment of Post Surgical Adhesions, pages 131–143

Interceed^R (TC7) AS AN ADJUVANT FOR ADHESION REDUCTION: ANIMAL STUDIES

Michael P. Diamond* Tim Cunningham** Cary B. Linsky** Lola Kamp** Robert F. McConnell,*** and Robert W Gracy****, *Division of Reproductive Endocrinology, Department of Obstetrics and Gynecology, Yale University School of Medicine, New Haven, CT,**Johnson & Johnson Patient Care, New Brunswick, NJ, ***Consultant Pathologist, Flemington, NJ, and ****Tissue Repair Unit, Department of Biochemistry, University of North Texas, Texas College of Osteopathic Medicine, Ft Worth, TX

INTRODUCTION

Interceed^R (TC7) is composed of oxidized regenerated cellulose in a special knitted weave. It is a distant cousin to Surgicel^R but differs in regard to the degree of oxidation, the porosity, the density, and the weave. Based on early observations that Surgicel^R was able to reduce adhesion development in some but not most animal models, (Diamond and DeCherney, 1987) the characteristics of Surgicel^R were altered in order to arrive at the final structure of Interceed^R (TC7). A variety of prototypes were identified and tested, with greatest efficacy for the prototype which came to be called Interceed^R (TC7). The differences between the woven pattern of Interceed^R (TC7) and Surgicel^R are depicted in Figure 1. The significance of this difference in the weave of the material will be alluded to later.

The initial animal efficacy studies were conducted in a rabbit uterine horn model (Linsky et al, 1987). The model consisted of performing a midline abdominal incision in the rabbit. The rabbit uterine horns were then exposed and a 5 cm segment of each horn scraped so as to initiate punctate bleeding. Bleeding was subsequently controlled by tamponade. If bleeding continued despite tamponade, the animal was excluded. After scraping both horns, the animal was then randomly assigned to either a control or treated group. In the treated group, the scraped section of each

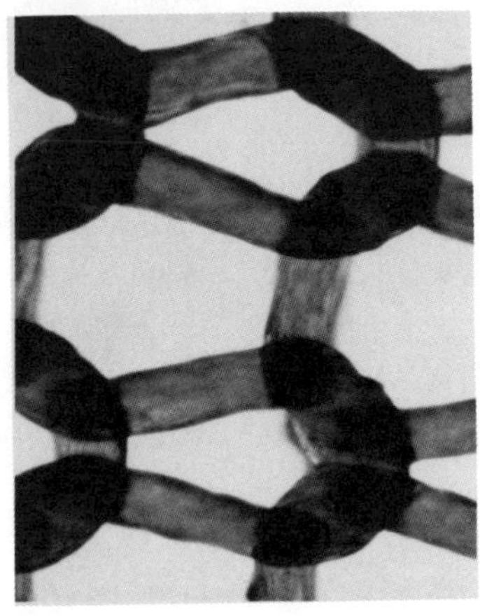

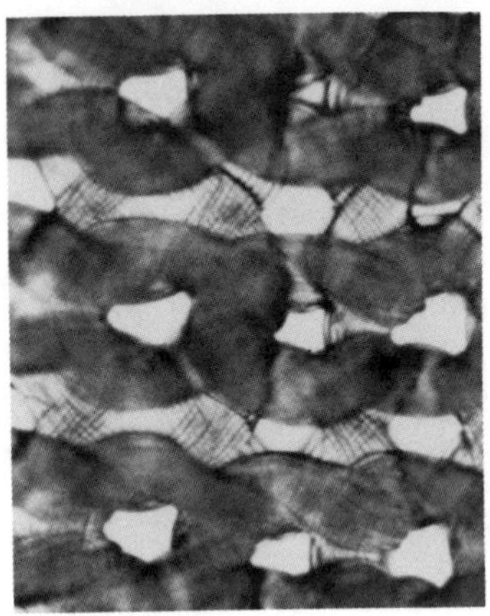

Surgicel®   Interceed® (TC7)

Figure 1 - Photos of weave of Surgicel® (left) and Interceed® (TC7) (right)

uterine horn as well as the underlying mesosalpinx was covered with a single sheet of Interceed® (TC7) and the material then moistened with saline. The abdomen was then closed with 3-0 vicryl suture and the skin with staples. Control and treated animals were necropsied 2, 4, and 8 weeks later by an observer unaware of the assignment group. Adhesions were scored on a 4 point maximum scoring system. As has been previously reported, treatment of the rabbit uterine horns with Interceed® (TC7) resulted in significant reduction in adhesion formation. The control rabbits had a mean score of 3.3±0.2/horn whereas those rabbits in which the horns were treated with Interceed® (TC7) had a mean score of 1.9±0.2 (Linsky et al, 1987). In comparison, the mean adhesion score in six rabbits treated with Surgicel®

(in the same manner as Interceed[R] (TC7) treatment) was 3.08±.24/horn. Thus, this study showed that Interceed[R] (TC7), was efficacious in reducing adhesions in this rabbit uterine horn model.

To further evaluate the efficacy in this material, a second rabbit model was devised (Diamond et al, 1987). This model was a sidewall model and allowed each animal to be its own control. The model consisted of excision of a 2X2 cm section of peritoneum on each sidewall, scraping a 2 cm segment of rabbit uterine horn adjacent to the sidewall lesion, and approximating the two lesioned areas with two 6-0 vicryl sutures outside the traumatized regions. Prior to completing approximation of the horn and sidewall, one side was randomly assigned to be treated with Interceed[R] (TC7). This was done in a picture frame fashion so as to overlap onto normal peritoneum. After placement, the material was moistened. Two weeks later, these animals were autopsied and adhesion scoring was performed by a blinded observer. The scoring system is based on a maximum score of 11. The mean adhesion score on the control sidewall was 9.0±0.3 which was significantly higher than the mean score on the Interceed[R] (TC7) treated sidewall of 6.8±0.4 (Diamond et al, 1987). Thus, in this model in which each animal served as its own control, Interceed[R] (TC7) was again identified to be effective in reducing adhesion formation.

Potential advantages of this biodegradable material are that it is easy to apply, that it remains in place without requiring suturing, and that it is able to be molded to the anatomical site to which it is to be applied. Questions that thus remained were the histological tissue response to this material, and the manner by which this material is metabolized.

Prior to discussion of these parameters, it is appropriate to describe the fate of the material after it is left in place on the peritoneal surface. As shown in Figure 2, after Interceed[R] (TC7) is applied to the peritoneal surface, it gelates such that after approximately eight hours, it has formed a continuous surface. Thus in this fashion, it is able to form a potential barrier between two otherwise apposing surfaces. In this way, it may be able to prevent and minimize the deposition of fibrin bands between these opposing surfaces, thereby preventing subsequent fibroblast ingrowth into the fibrin mass, and thus the

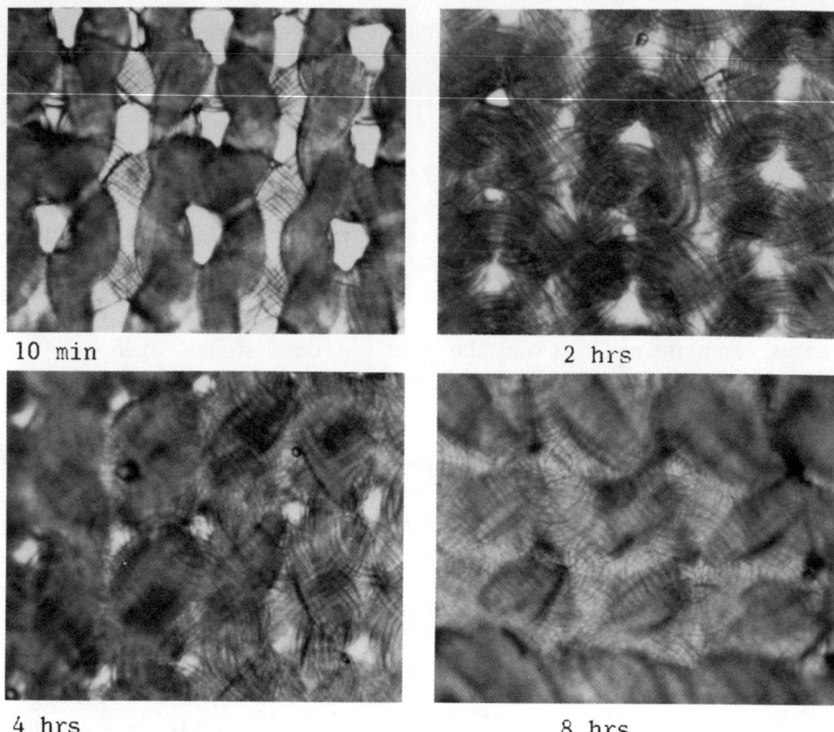

Figure 2 - Gelation sequence of Interceed[R] (TC7) after placement for 10 minutes, two hours, four hours, and eight hours.

generation of adhesions. While this hypothesis remains only a theory as to the mechanism of action of this material, it seems plausible based on all of the data available at this time.

Histological response of peritoneal surfaces to Interceed[R] (TC7) has been evaluated at multiple time points after placement to the material. Macroscopically, the material appears to be nearly all gone by approximately 3-4 days. Its metabolism does not typically elicit production of foreign body giant cells which are frequently observed with other biological implants (Figure 3). The degree of inflammation was not different from that of the scraped but untreated control rabbit uterine horns. The appearance of the Interceed[R] (TC7) treated peritoneal surface was difficult to distinguish from untreated peritoneum after 20 days. Figure 3 shows micrographs of peritoneum from treated and untreated sidewalls at 4, 14, and 28 days after treatment. The primary cellular response identified is that of mononuclear macrophages. There was no histomorphological evidence that Interceed[R] (TC7) was detrimental to macrophage physiology.

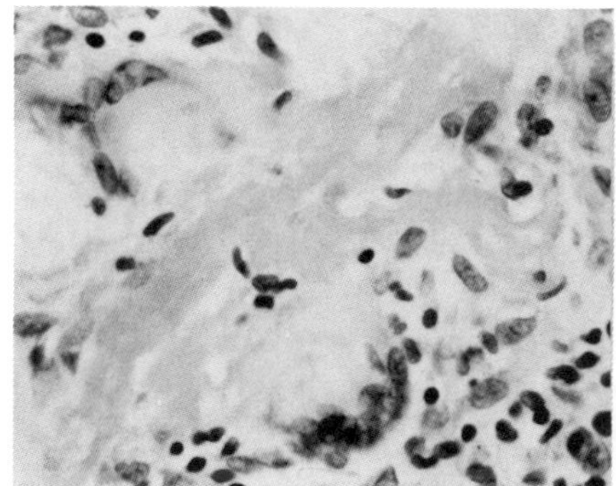

Figure 3A

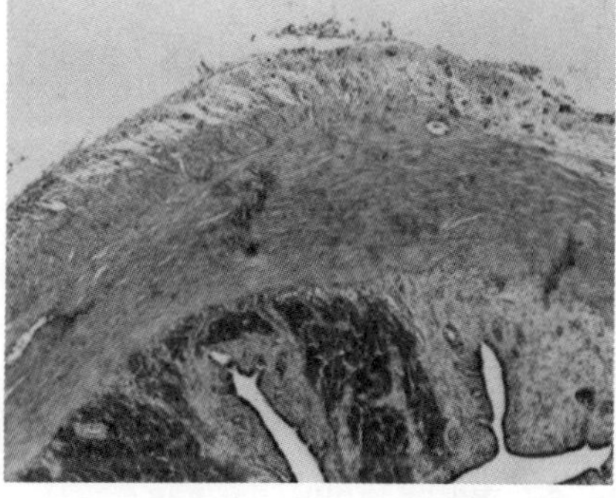

Figure 3B

Figure 3-A. Cellular response to collagen characterized by foreign body giant cell reaction.

B.Interceed[R] (TC7) <u>DAY 4</u> H&E 40X-Uterine horn showing roughened peritoneal surface (serosal surface) damage and covered with Interceed[R] (TC7). Note the lack of any significant fibroblastic or inflammatory cell activity. The endometrial stromal hemorrhage is secondary to surgical manipulation.

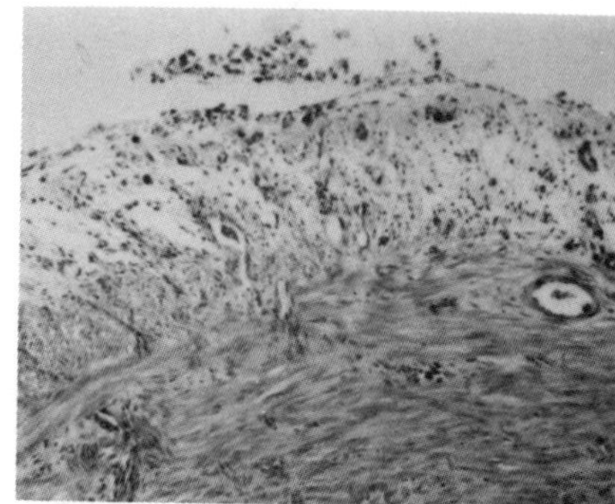

Figure 3C

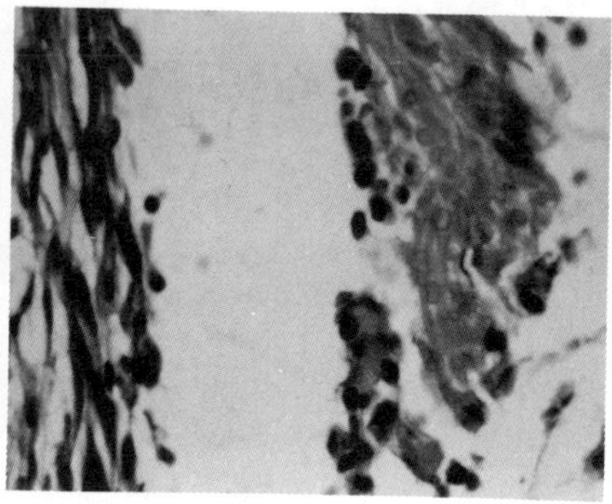

Figure 3D

C. Interceed[R] (TC7) DAY 4 H&E 100X-Same section as above showing the redevelopment of the peritoneal covering. A few mononuclear macrophages in the region where Interceed[R] (TC7) was located. Mild edema and new vessels are present beneath the peritoneal surface.

D. Interceed[R] (TC7) DAY 4 H&E 400X-A high power view of a small amount of Interceed[R] (TC7) (dark pink material) mixed with a few erythrocytes. Note the typical mononuclear macrophage activity. The cytoplasm of some appear to contain pink Interceed[R] (TC7) material. There is a slight fibroblastic response at the myometrial surface.

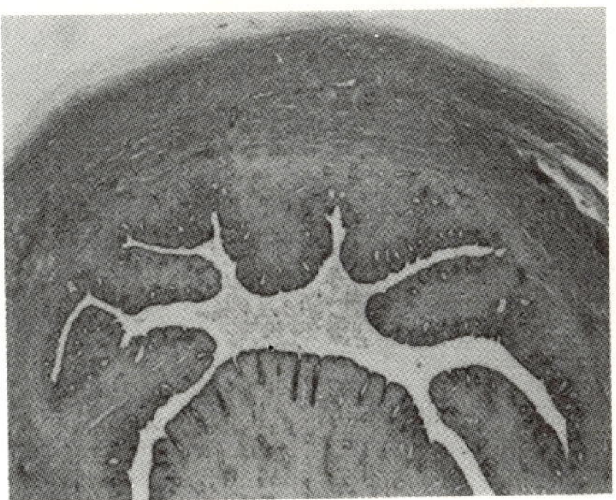

Figure 3E

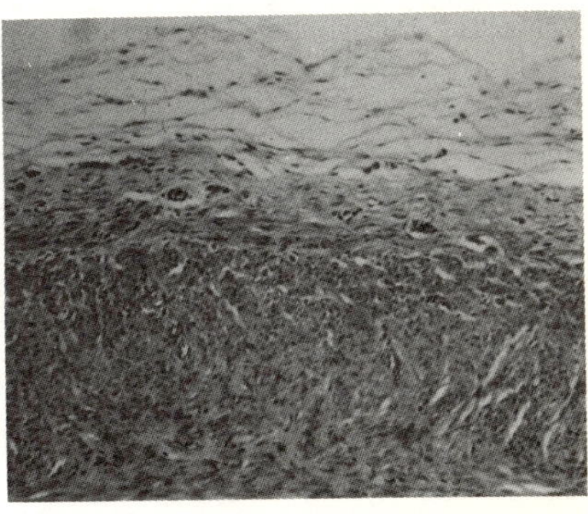

Figure 3F

E. Interceed[R] (TC7) DAY 14
H&E 16X-Macroscopic photo showing the lack of fibrous adhesions over the peritoneal surface of the horn. There is only a slight proliferation of the peritoneal covering which is complete by day 14.

F. Interceed[R] (TC7) DAY 14
100X-The peritoneal (serosal) surface is intact and without cellular reaction or fibrous tags or adhesions.

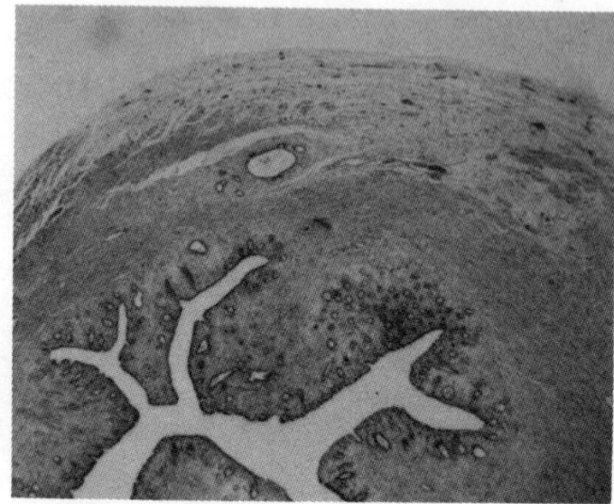

Figure 3G

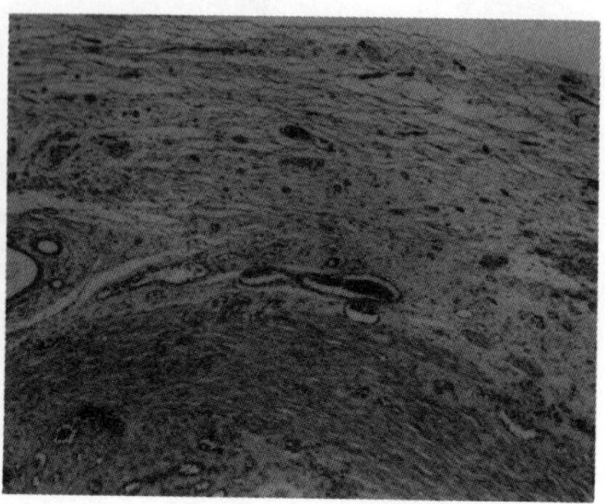

Figure 3H

G. Interceed[R] (TC7) 1 MONTH
16X-A macroscopic photo of the uterine horn showing a segment of the outer myometrial wall with a large surgical lesion would normally result in omental or sidewall adhesions if left unaided. The defect has been filled with loose connective tissue.

H. Interceed[R] (TC7) 1 MONTH
40X-A higher power view of the damaged area showing the orderly filling with loose connection tissue and new vessels. Note the lack of fibrous tags at the surface.

The histological findings are very consistent with that obtained from studies of the in vivo and in vitro metabolism of Interceed[R] (TC7) (Dimitrijevich et al, In Press; Dimitrijevich et al, In Press). The molecular structure of cellulose and oxidized regenerated cellulose is shown in Figure 4. The difference is conversion of the primary hydroxyl group (CH_2OH on carbon 6) to a carboxyl group. This oxidation makes the β1-4 linkages susceptible to both hydrolysis and enzymatic cleavage. This linkage is now a potential substrate for degradation by macrophages which contain lysosomal hydrolytic enzymes (β1-4 glucosidase and β1-4 glucuronidase) which cleave the β1-4 linkages.

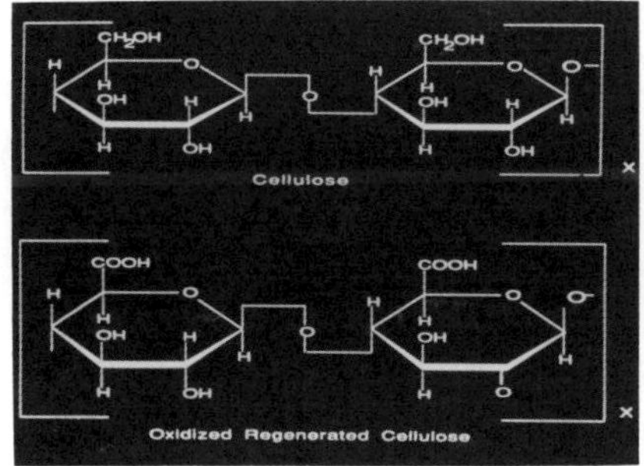

Figure 4

Figure 4 - Structure of cellulose and its oxidation products, oxidized regenerated cellulose, which compose Interceed[R] (TC7).

In vitro and in vivo studies examining metabolism of Interceed[R] (TC7) have been performed (Dimitrijevich et al, In Press; Dimitrijevich et al, In Press). The in vivo studies consisted of lavage of the peritoneal cavity at variable times after placement of the material with subsequent analysis of the in vivo breakdown products as a function of time. The in vivo degradation products were the same as previously identified from in vitro studies (Dimitrijevich et al, In Press). The degradation products suggest that Interceed[R] (TC7) is degraded by a chain shortening process which yields oligosaccharides, with subsequent metabolism to glucuronic acid and glucose which are able to be handled through well defined metabolic pathways. Analysis of the lavage fluids at timed intervals after placement of the Interceed[R] (TC7) is shown in Figure 5. These figures demonstrate that the molecular size and

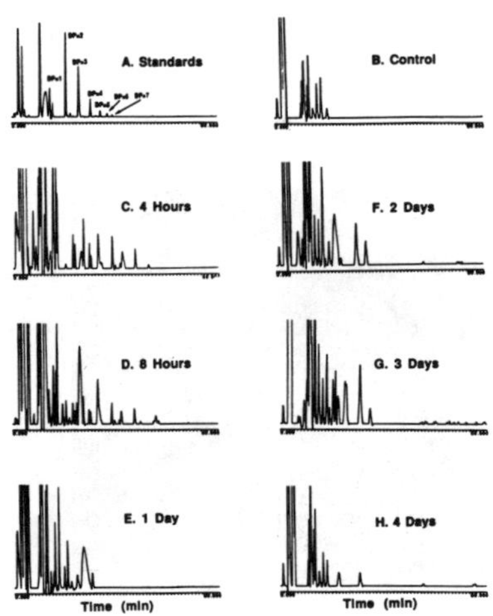

Figure 5 - H.p.l.c. - p.a.d chromatograms of rabbit peritoneal lavages showing kinetics of bio-degradation of Interceed[R] (TC7) and clearance of the resulting oligosaccharides. A. Oligomers of D-galacturonic acid (D.P. =degree of polymerisation); B. Typical lavage from control animals; C-H. Lavages from test animals taken at 4 and 8 hours and 1,2,3 and 4 days after implantation of Interceed[R] (TC7).

quantity of oligomeric products begin to decline during the first day after placement. With increasing time, the oligomers become shorter and of lesser quantity. By four days, essentially only short chain oligosaccharides remain. Since the degradation products did not accumulate in either blood or serum, a local intraperitoneal clearance of Interceed® (TC7) is suggested. Furthermore, these biochemical changes, and the time course over which they occur coincides with the histological findings that the Interceed® (TC7) was rarely identified after four days intraabdominally.

Peritoneal macrophages are involved in the clearance of foreign material from the peritoneal cavity. Involvement of macrophages in metabolism of Interceed® (TC7) was demonstrated by reaction of the glucuronic acid metabolites with lead acetate. The lead acetate complex was subsequently able to be identified within macrophages by x-ray emission during scanning electron microscopy, and in thin sections during transmission electron microscopy (Figure 6). This electromicrograph demonstrates a macrophage with labeled fragments of Interceed® (TC7) identified within lysosomes (which contain the β-glycosidase and β-glucuronidase required for further degradation of Interceed® (TC7).

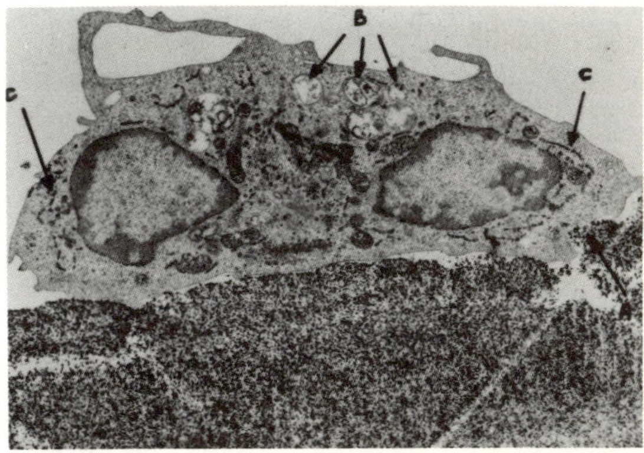

Figure 6 - Scanning Electron Microgram (S.E.M.) of a rabbit peritoneal macrophage exposed to lead labeled Interceed®(TC7) (total magnification 8,220x). Arrow at A shows ingestion of Interceed®; Arrows at B show degradation of the material within the intercellular vacuoles; Arrows at C show lead label associated with some of the cellular membranes.

Several other observations have been made which have potential impact on clinical application in the use of Interceed[R] (TC7). First, it is essential that meticulous hemostasis be achieved prior to application of the material. If the blood saturates oxidized regenerated cellulose, the ability of this material to reduce adhesion formation is ameliorated (Linsky et al, 1988). Secondly, the resorption of the material within the body is dependent on the surface contact of the material with intraabdominal surfaces. This is evidenced by the observation that layers of Interceed[R] (TC7) on opposing peritoneal surfaces will require longer time periods to be absorbed. Consequently, if the material becomes folded or "balled up", it would be anticipated that the material would persist for longer periods of time.

In summary, these animal models demonstrate that Interceed[R] (TC7) significantly reduces postoperative adhesion formation. The material is resorbed by the body, presumably by intraperitoneal processes over a very short time, and without evidence of typical foreign body reaction. As described later in this book by Russell Malinak, efficacy of Interceed[R] (TC7) in reducing postoperative adhesion reformation has now been demonstrated in human clinical trials. Future research efforts will assess whether further improvement in the efficacy of Interceed[R] (TC7) can be achieved by application of pharmacologic agents to the barrier.

REFERENCES

Diamond MP, DeCherney AH (1987). Pathogenesis of adhesion formation/ reformation: Application to Reproductive Surgery. Microsurgery 8:103-107.

Diamond MP, Linsky CB, Cunningham T, Constantine B, DeCherney AH (1986). Reduction of adhesion formation with TC7, an absorbable biocompatible barrier: efficacy of double wrap. XII World Congress on Fertility and Sterility, Singapore, October.

Diamond MP, Linsky CB, Cunningham T, Constantine B, diZerega GS, DeCherney AH (1987). Development of a model for sidewall adhesions in the rabbit and their reduction by an absorbable barrier. Microsurgery 8:197-200.

Dimitrijevich SD, Tatarko M, Gracy RW, Linsky CB, Olsen C: Biodegradation of oxidized regenerated cellulose. Carbohydrate Research. In Press.

Dimitrìjevich SD, Tatarko M, Gracy RW, Wise GE, Oakford LX, Linsky CB, Kamp L: In vivo degradation of oxidized regenerated cellulose. Carbohydrate Research. In Press.

Linsky CB, Diamond MP, Cunningham T, Constantine B, DeCherney AH, diZerega GS (1987). Adhesion reduction in a rabbit uterine horn model using TC-7. J Reprod Med 32:17-20.

Linsky CB, Diamond MP, Cunningham T, DeCherney AH, diZerega G (1988). Effect of blood on the efficacy of barrier adhesion reduction in the rabbit uterine horn model. Infertility 11:273-280.

Treatment of Post Surgical Adhesions, pages 145–155

ALTERNATIVE REPRODUCTIVE TECHNOLOGIES VS. ADHESIOLYSIS

William R. Meyer, Alan H. DeCherney

Division of Reproductive Endocrinology, Yale University School of Medicine, Department of Obstetrics and Gynecology, New Haven, CT 06510

INTRODUCTION

The second annual report of the in vitro fertilization (IVF) Registry noted a surge in the number of stimulation cycles from 2,864 in 1986 to 14,647 in 1987 (Medical Research International et al, 1989). As a consequence, the public has generally become more aware of the various aspects of assisted reproductive technology. To the ten percent of couples misfortuned with infertility this five fold increase in stimulation cycles might easily be misinterpreted as representing increasing pregnancy rates. Fortunately the Registry report is quick to point out that four of the 96 IVF clinics were responsible for one-third of all clinical pregnancies conceived through IVF. In addition, the Registry notes that the clinical pregnancy rate for IVF-embryo transfer (ET) during this time frame has remained constant at sixteen percent (Medical Research International et al, 1989).

These percentages are of obvious importance to women afflicted with tuboperitoneal adhesive disease, as figures reflecting GIFT (gamete intrafallopian transfer), ZIFT (zygote intrafallopian transfer), and TPET (tubal pre-embryo transfer) success rates are of little relevance to their problem. Unfortunately IVF-ET is often perceived as the final opportunity for a couples attempts at conception and parenthood. Persistent frustration frequently results in premature enrollment into a IVF-ET program without full consideration of other full options including surgery. Up to date experience with results of tubal microsurgery and in vitro fertilization allows physicians the ability to provide information and appropriate counseling for women with various degrees of tuboperitoneal adhesive disease. This allows advice directed towards optimal chances of pregnancy whether the avenue pursued be adhesiolysis, salpingostomy, fimbrioplasty, balloon tuboplasty or in vitro fertilization embryo transfer.

ADHESIOLYSIS VS IVF-ET

Tubal corrective surgery and adhesiolysis have been the main stay for the treatment of tuboperitoneal adhesive disease. Adhesiolysis has traditionally been accomplished by sharp scissor dissection and/or electrocautery. Recently these two modalities have been commonly replaced by the laser. However when the carbon dioxide laser was compared to electromicrosurgery, the two were equally effective in adhesiolysis (Pittaway et al, 1983; Filmar et al, 1986). A comparative histological evaluation of tissue healing after use of these three modalities demonstrated the most extensive foreign body reaction subsequent to use of the microelectrode (Filmar et al, 1989; Filmar et al, 1989). Sharp mechanical dissection resulted in the least amount of tissue necrosis and was recommended as the modality of choice. This histological data has failed to be substantiated by increased pregnancy rates or reduced adhesion formation when the carbon dioxide laser is compared to electromicrocautery (Tulandi, 1986). Still the laser continues to be the instrument of choice for most infertility surgeons.

The necessity of magnification during adhesiolysis is no better established than is the inherent value of either the laser, scissors or electrocautery. Intuitively magnification would seem to facilitate the differentiation of adhesion-peritoneal interfaces while embodying the other basic tenets of micro surgery. Diamond reported that microsurgical gynecologic salpingolysis afforded a 2-fold increase in term pregnancy rates when compared to the microsurgical approach (Diamond, 1979). Other investigators using the conventional technique have demonstrated similar term pregnancy rates in comparison to microsurgery. (See Table 1)

TABLE 1. Conventional (Macro) versus Microsurgical lysis of adhesions.

	No. of patients	% live births
Conventional Technique		
Bronson and Wallach	35	57
Spadoni	8	75
Diamond	220	25
Caspi and Halperin	101	46
Betz et al	29	69
Microsurgery		
Diamond	140	57
Luber et al	13	62
Frantzen and Schlösser	49	39
Hulka	47	26
Tulandi	33	52
Donnez and Cusanas Roux	42	64

Endoscopic adhesiolysis is rapidly becoming the modern operative approach to this disease process (Luciano et al, 1989) confirmed clinical conjecture that laparoscopic laser surgery is effective in reducing intraperitoneal adhesions and it results in less postoperative adhesion formation than does laparotomy. Both Fayez (Fayez, 1983) and Gomel (Gomel, 1983) report live birth pregnancy rates following laparoscopic lysis of adhesions comparable to results at laparotomy. Unfortunately the destructive effects of adhesive disease are rarely limited to the peritoneal surface and direct comparisons and interpretation of these published studies remains difficult. Regardless of this fact the term intrauterine pregnancy rate following adhesiolysis exceeds those associated with in vitro fertilization-embryo transfer and the latter should not be considered unless severe tubal compromise is coexistent.

COMPLETE DISTAL TUBAL OBSTRUCTION: SURGERY VS IVF

Neosalpingostomy, the creation of a new tubal ostium, has been the accepted method of treatment of distal tubal occlusion. Concurrently the success of IVF-ET has established itself as a viable alternative to neosalpingostomy in selected cases. Although post neosalpingostomy tubal patency rates approximate 90-95%, pregnancy rates are at best one-third the patency rate. Winston (Winston, 1981) reviewed a series of 653 macroscopic salpingostomies and compared this to a series of 324 microsurgical salpingostomies. He concluded that microsurgical neosalpingostomy resulted in a significantly increased intrauterine pregnancy rate. However O'Brien and co-workers report a 25% pregnancy rate following macroscopic neosalpingostomy (O'Brien, 1969). Hence, a clear advantage of microsurgery for neosalpingostomy seems lacking. More recently several reports of endoscopic salpingostomy have been published (Fayez, 1983; Daniell et al, 1984; Diamond et al, 1986). In comparison to laparotomy these results from laparoscopy appear suboptimal, but this may reflect the selection of two distinct patient populations.

Several factors influence the success of neosalpingostomy for distal tubal occlusion. Depressed pregnancy rates are reflective of probable intraluminal tubal pathology and little evidence exists to support that regenerative mucosal changes occur after patency is established (Winston, 1981). Rock et al reviewed 87 patients who underwent neosalpingostomy (Rock et al, 1978). Pregnancy rates were compared to the extent of adjoining adhesive disease, tubal thickness and diameter, along with hysterosalpingographic findings. (Table 2)

TABLE 2. Rock Classification of the Extent of Tubal Disease with Distal Tubal Obstruction

Extent of Disease	Findings
Mild	Absent or small hydrosalpinx ≤15 mm diameter Inverted fimbria easily recognized when patency achieved No significant peritubal or periovarian adhesions Preoperative hysterogram reveals a rugal pattern
Moderate	Hydrosalpinx 15–30 mm diameter Fragments of fimbria not readily identified Periovarian and/or peritubal adhesions without fixation, minimal cul-de-sac adhesions Absence of rugal pattern on preoperative hysterogram
Severe	Large hydrosalpinx ≥ 30 mm diameter No fimbria Dense pelvic or adnexal adhesions with fixation of the ovary and tube to either the broad ligament, pelvic sidewall, omentum, and/or bowel Obliteration of the cul-de-sac Frozen pelvis(adhesion formation so dense that limits of organs are difficult to define)

More recently Boer-Meisel et al (Boer-Meisel et al, 1986) prospectively analyzed similar associated factors and reported their predictive value of post neosalpingostomy intrauterine and ectopic pregnancy rates in 108 women. The results were similar to Rock's retrospective study (Table 3). Interestingly the diameter of the hydrosalpinx in the prospective analysis did not correlate with the prediction of subsequent pregnancy. Tuboscopy and fimbrial biopsy may assist in determination of postoperative pregnancy rates (Donnez et al, 1986; Shapiro et al, 1988; Broyne et al, 1989).

TABLE 3. Classification of hydrosalpinx and resultant postoperative pregnancy rates.

	Pregnancies	Severe (%)	Moderate (%)	Mild(%)
	intrauterine	5	17	80
Rock et al	ectopic	0	13	6
	intrauterine	3	21	77
Boer-Meisel	ectopic	16	27	4
et al	miscarriage	0	5	19

It seems reasonable to compare these results with those of the 1987 IVF Registry in attempts to determine the treatment of choice in women with distal tubal obstruction. Women with mild distal tubal total occlusive disease would have to undergo 5-6 oocyte retrievals to attain similar success to surgery. Interestingly the reported IVF-ET ectopic rate of seven percent in IVF-ET is comparable to surgical results in women with mild hydrosalpingeal disease (Medical Research International et al, 1989).

With moderate distal total occlusive disease post neosalpingostomy, similar intrauterine pregnancy rates can be obtained after 1 retrieval cycle of IVF-ET. In addition the ectopic rate of 13-27% postoperatively favors IVF-ET for women with this degree of tubal disease (Medical Research International et al, 1989).

The advantage of IVF-ET for women with severe hydrosalpingeal tubal disease is readily apparent. One transfer cycle of IVF-ET offers the couple a four times greater chance of having an intrauterine pregnancy (Medical International et al, 1989).

When debating over a surgical or a non-surgical avenue in patients with distal occlusive disease the physician should not only be aware of these figures, but should be cognizant of the fact that a twenty five percent risk of miscarriage occurs through IVF-ET.

INCOMPLETE DISTAL TUBAL OBSTRUCTION: FIMBRIOPLASTY VS IVF

Various degrees of tubal pathology contributing to partial distal occlusion make interpretation and comparison of postoperative success rates in this group the most difficult. A summary of pregnancy outcome following fimbrioplasty is presented in Table 4.

TABLE 4. Pregnancy Outcome Subsequent to Fimbrioplasty

Microsurgical	No. of patients	% pregnant	%ectopic pregnant
Frantzen and Schlösser	49	22.4	4.1
Patton	40	63.0	5.0
Donnez and Casanas-Roux	132	60.0	2.0
Luber	21	25.0	9.5
Conventional			
Wallach et al	24	20.8	8.1
Young et al	24	25.0	8.1
Trimbos-Kemper et al	52	51.0	N/A

Values with either conventional or microscopic fimbroiplasty remain intermediary between those results obtained subsequent to neosalpingostomy and adhesiolysis. All values exceed the percentage success rate obtained with one retrieval or transfer cycle (18%) of IVF-ET (Medical International et al, 1989). Fimbrioplasty should remain the primary mode of therapy for incomplete distal tubal occlusion with IVF-ET reserved for those patients failing to attain pregnancy during a predetermined period post fimbrioplasty. The length of time appropriated for natural conception would vary based on the severity of the tubal disease, associated infertility factors, patient age, and financial constraints.

PROXIMAL TUBAL DISEASE: SURGERY VS IVF

Occlusion of the proximal oviductal segment can result from endometriosis, tubal sterilization, or infection. Among tubal operations, 20% are devoted to correction of interstitial tubal obstruction. Tubouterine implantation techniques have been replaced by microsurgical tubocornual anastomosis, allowing preservation of the physiologic function of the uterotubal junction; tubal length and vascular integrity. After the procedure, whether the initial insult was infection or sterilization, various authors have reported intrauterine pregnancy rates in excess of 50%, with ectopic pregnancy rates approximating 8-12% (Patton et al, 1986; Lavy et al, 1986; Gillett et al, 1989). Recently, transcervical balloon tuboplasty under fluoroscopic guidance, has been used to "unocclude" cases of proximal obstruction. Although pregnancy rates have failed to approach anastomotic success, the procedure remains new and is obviously associated with less morbidity. Reocclusion rates, along with both intrauterine and ectopic pregnancy rates need to be determined prior to its routine use as an alternative to microsurgery (Confino et al, 1988).

Based on current publication microsurgical tubo-cornual anastomosis remains the treatment of choice for well documented interstitial tubal occlusion. Balloon tuboplasty may eventually play an integral part in the treatment of this disease. Presently IVF-ET should be reserved for cases of surgical failure.

CONCLUSION

The goal of adhesiolysis and various tuboplastic procedures is simply to facilitate fertilization and provide passage of the zygote into the uterus. If the chances of success are greater extracorporeally, then IVF-ET should be the treatment of choice in place of surgery. Less often are the two procedures used in combination (Roh et al, 1988). Adhesiolysis is rarely indicated for the purpose of augmenting ovarian folliculogenesis prior to IVF-ET as adhesions have been found to have no deleterious effect on ovarian function (Diamond et al, 1988). In addition transvaginal sonographic oocyte retrieval has all but obviated the need for pelvic reconstructive surgery designed to facilitate endoscopic ovarian access. Unfortunately the decision of whether to pursue IVF-ET or gynecologic surgery is never straight forward. In addition, intangibles including the patient's age, third party payment reimbursement and neighboring IVF program and surgeon success rates will influence the final decision. Unfortunately Wood and Trounson's suggestion that in vitro fertilization and embryo transfer may be preferred to tubal surgery if the expected success rate of the latter is less than three laparoscopic retrievals-may already be obsolete (Wood et al, 1984). Trans vaginal sonographic oocyte retrievals, embryo co-culturing, perizona pellucida drilling in IVF-ET; along with the introduction of new surgical modalities designed to reduce adhesions, balloon tuboplasty and new laser modalities will continue to further modify Wood and Trounson's recommendations.

REFERENCES

Betz G, Engel T, Penney LL (1980). Tuboplasty: comparison of the methodology. Fertil Steril 34:534-36.

Boer-Meisel ME, te Velde ER, Habbema JDF, Kardaun JW (1986). Predicting the pregnancy outcome in patients treated for hydrosalpinx: a prospective study. Fertil Steril 45:23-29.

Bronson RA, Wallach EE (1977). Lysis of periadnexal adhesion for correction of infertility. Fertil Steril 28:613-19.

Broyne FD, Puttemans P, Boeckx W, Brosens I (1989). The clinical value of salpingoscopy in tubal infertility. Fertil Steril 51:339-40.

Caspi E, Halperin Y, Bukovsky I (1979). The importance of periadnexal adhesions in tubal reconstructive surgery for infertility. Fertil Steril 31:296-304.

Confino E, Friberg J, Gleicher N (1988) Preliminary experience with transcervical balloon tuboplasty. Am J Obstet Gynecol 159:370-5.

Daniell JF, Herbert CM (1984). Laparoscopic salpingostomy utilizing the CO_2 laser. Fertil Steril 41:558-63.

Diamond MP, Pellicer A, Boyers SP, DeCherney AH (1988). The effect of periovarian adhesion follicular development in patients undergoing ovarian stimulation for in vitro fertilization-embryo transfer. Fertil Steril (49:100-103).

Diamond MP, DeCherney AH, Polan ML (1986) Laparoscopic use of the argon laser in non-endometriotic reproductive pelvic surgery. J Reprod Med 31:1101-1105.

Diamond E (1979). Lysis of post-operative adhesions in infertility. Fertil Steril 31:287-95.

Donnez J, Casanas-Roux F (1986). Prognostic factors of fimbrial microsurgery. Fertil Steril 46:200-204.

Fayez JA (1983). An assessment of the role of operative laparoscopy in tuboplasty. Fertil Steril 39:476-479.

Filmar S, Jetha N, McComb P, Gomel V (1989). A comparative histologic study on the healing process after tissue transection. Carbon dioxide laser and surgical microscissors. Am J Obstet Gynecol 160:1068-72.

Filmar S, Jetha N, McComb P, Gomel V (1989). A comparative histologic study on the healing process after tissue transection. Carbon dioxide laser and electro microsurgery. Am J Obstet Gynecol 160:1062-7.

Filmar S, Gomel V, McComb P (1986). The effectiveness of CO_2 laser and electro microsurgery adhesiolysis: a comparative study. Fertil Steril 45:489-491.

Frantzen C, Schlosser HW (1982). Microsurgery and post infectious tubal infertility. Fertil Steril 38:397-402.

Gillett WR, Herbison GP (1989). Tubocornual anastomosis: surgical considerations and coexistent infertility factors in determining the prognosis. Fertil Steril 51:241-246.

Gomel N (1983). Salpingo-ovariolysis by laparoscopy in infertility. Fertil Steril 40:607-611.

Hulka JF (1982). Adnexal adhesions: a prognostic staging and classifications system based on a five-year survey of fertility surgery results at Chapel Hill, North Carolina. Am J Obstet Gynecol 144:141-47.

Lavy G, Diamond MP, DeCherney AH (1986). Pregnancy following tubocornual anastomosis. Fertil Steril 46:21-25.

Luber K, Beeson CC, Kennedy JF, Villanueva B, Young PE (1986). Results of microsurgical treatment of tubal infertility and early second look laparoscopy in the post-pelvic inflammatory disease patient: implications for in-vitro fertilization. Am J Obstet Gynecol 145:1264-70.

Luciano AA, Maier DB, Koch EI, Nulsen JC, Whitman GF (1989). A comparative study of postoperative adhesions following laser surgery by laparoscopy versus laparotomy in the rabbit model. Obstet Gynecol 74:220-24.

Medical Research International and the Society of Assisted Reproductive Technology, (1989). In Vitro Fertilization/Embryo Transfer in the United States: 1987 results from the National IVF-ET Registry. Fertil Steril 51:13-18.

O'Brien Jr, Arronet GH, Eduljee SYA (1969). Operative treatment of fallopian tube pathology in human fertility. Am J Obstet Gynecol 103:520-526.

Patton PP, William JJ, Coulam CB (1986). Microsurgical reconstruction of the proximal oviduct. Fertil Steril 47:35-39.

Patton GW Jr (1982). Pregnancy outcome following microsurgical fimbrioplasty. Fertil Steril 37:150-55.

Pittaway DE, Maxson WS, Daniell JF (1983). A comparison of the CO_2 laser and electrocautery on postoperative intraperitoneal adhesion formation in rabbits. Fertil Steril 40:366-68.

Rock JA, Kata Yama KP, Martin EJ, Woodruff JD, Jones HH (1978). Factors influencing the success of salpingostomy techniques for distal fimbrial obstruction. Obstet Gynecol 52:591-596.

Roh SI, Dodds WG, Park JM, Awadulla SG, Friedman CI, Kim MH (1988). In vitro fertilization with concurrent pelvic reconstructive surgery. Fertil Steril 49:96-99.

Shapiro BS, Diamond MP, DeCherney AH (1988). Salpingoscopy: an adjunctive technique for evaluation of the fallopian tube. Fertil Steril 49:1076-9.

Spandoni LR (1980). Tubal and peritubal surgery without magnification: an analysis. Am J Obstet Gynecol 137:189-195.

Trimbos-Kemper TCM, Trimbos JB, van Hall EV (1985). Adhesions formation after tubal surgery: results of eighth day laparoscopy in 188 patients. Fertil Steril 43:395-400.

Tulandi T (1986). Salpingo-ovaviolysis: a comparison between laser surgery and electrosurgery. Fertil Steril 45:489-491.

Wallach EE, Manara LR, Eisenberg E (1983). Experience with 143 cases of tubal surgery. Fertil Steril 39:609-617.

Winston RML (1981) Is microsurgery a necessity for salpingostomy? The evaluation of results. Aust NZJ Obstet Gynecol 21:143-152.

Wood C, Trounson A (1984). Clinical In Vitro Fertilization. Springer-Verlag New York.

Young PE, Egan JE, Barlow JJ, Milligan WJ (1970). Reconstructive surgery for infertility at the Boston Hospital for women. Am J Obstet Gynecol 108:1092-97.

Treatment of Post Surgical Adhesions, pages 157–163

Dextran 70--Encouraging Early Clinical Studies

Sanford M. Rosenberg, M.D., Director

Richmond Center for Fertility and Endocrinology, Ltd.
7605 Forest Avenue Suite 207
Richmond, Virginia 23229

INTRODUCTION

With the increasing understanding that no single surgical or medical adjuvant was wholly useful in the management or prevention of surgical adhesions, the search continued in the early 1980's for a more "universal" modality to effect improvement. At that time significant enthusiasm developed for the use of high molecular weight dextran-70 in the prevention of adhesions. This was based largely on encouraging data from animal studies in several species including rabbits (Neuwirth and Khalaf 1975, Utian et al, 1979, Holtz et al, 1980), Rhesus monkeys (diZerega & Hodgen, 1980) and pigs (Luengo and van Hall 1978). Why was dextran-70 considered? Besides the encouraging animal data, there had been a demonstrated long history of safe intraperitoneal use via hysteroscopy, the compound was simple to use, relatively inexpensive, and very well tolerated with minimal side effects. In view of the relative benignity of the compound and its previous large-scale safe use, clinical usage in patients to treat and/or prevent adhesions became widespread before human data was available.

CONTROLLED HUMAN STUDIES

Two studies were designed to address this issue: The Adhesion Study Group, coordinated by the Pregnancy Research Branch of the National Institute of Child Health and Human Development (Fertil Steril 40:612,

1983) and Rosenberg & Board (Am J Obstet Gynecol 148:380, 1984). Both studies were randomized prospective and double blinded. Both evaluated adhesions at a primary laparotomy and then re-evaluated them within three months at a second-look laparoscopy. Differences between the two studies were relatively minor. The Adhesion Study Group involved the use of 250 ml. of dextran-70, in 55 patients, and used 250 ml. of normal saline as a control in 47 patients. Rosenberg and Board used a volume of 200 ml. of dextran-70 in 23 patients and 200 ml. of Ringers lactate as control in 21 patients. The Adhesion Study Group used a modification of the adhesion scoring system of Hulka et al (1978), and the Rosenberg and Board study utilized the adhesion scoring system associated with the American Fertility Society classification of Endometriosis forms.

In all cases, strict attention was paid to standard microsurgical technique including careful handling of tissue with fine, atraumatic instruments, meticulous hemostasis with bipolar or microneedle unipolar cautery, use of fine caliber non-reactive sutures, and constant irrigation with body temperature irrigating solutions. Operating microscopes were used wherever appropriate, including all tubal procedures. All patients in both studies were given a short course (1-3 doses) of single-agent prophylactic antibiotics. No other adjuvant therapies including steroids, antihistamines, or post-operative hydrotubations were used. All patients were initially evaluated at the time of the original laparotomy according to the individual scoring systems involved, and were re-evaluated by the original surgeons at the second look laparoscopy. All patients in the Rosenberg and Board study maintained protected intercourse until after the laparoscopy, although this was not true in the Adhesion Study Group protocol.

The multicenter Adhesion Study Group found that in 102 patients dextran-70 "effectively" reduced post operative adhesion formation and that "patients with a marked reduction in adhesion formation... were found to occur more frequently in the [dextran-70] group (... $p<0.05$)".

Rosenberg and Board, in their 44 patients, demonstrated "a significant difference ($p=0.016$) between the two groups with respect to the net change in adhesion scores overall, with dextran-70 treated patients demonstrating much greater improvement." Further, in those patients undergoing lysis of pre-existing adhesions, the overall improvement in adhesion scores of the dextran-70 group was "even more obvious" ($p<0.05$).

The Adhesion Study Group also noted that the adhesion reduction effect appeared to be limited to those patients with "severe" adhesions initially ($p<0.025$). Both studies noted that the effect was largely limited to "dependent" portions of the pelvis. This was actually quantitated by the Adhesion Study Group study and noted as a subjective observation in the Rosenberg and Board study. Both sets of investigators, therefore, demonstrated that they had observed demonstrable, statistically significant efficacy of high molecular weight dextran, and these studies were used--and continue to be used--to justify the use of these agents, particularly in those situations where adhesion formation or reformation is clinically expected.

DISCUSSION

Dextran is a chain polysaccharide derivative of sugar beets. It is very viscous and the 70,000 molecular weight variety is very slowly absorbed from the peritoneal cavity with over 50% being present in the peritoneum for 7-10 days (Polishuk and Bercovici, 1971). Shwartzkopff (1965) found that the rate of transfer of dextran-70 across peritoneal membranes in humans was only 1.2% of that of water. For this reason, high molecular weight dextran, slowly absorbed across peritoneal membranes, produces an osmotic gradient in the peritoneal cavity resulting in a transient ascites. Dextran 40, on the other hand, with a molecular weight of 40,000, appears to be absorbed within 24 hours. This may account for the multiple reports of the ineffectiveness of this latter agent in reducing adhesions (deZerega and Hodgen, 1980, Seitz et al, 1973, Polishuk and Bercovici, 1971).

Two major theories have been proposed to account for the mechanism of action of high molecular weight dextran. Dextran-70 is known to facilitate the lysis of fibrin (Tangen et al, 1972, Wallenbeck and Tangen 1975, and Misirlioglu and Shafiroff, 1973) both *in vivo* and *in vitro*. In view of the well known significance of fibrin deposition in the formation of post-operative adhesions, dextran may reduce adhesion formation by directly promoting fibrinolysis.

A second theory, supported by the evidence that dextran-70's effect is greatest in dependent portions of the pelvis, is often referred to as the "osmotic", or "hydroflotation" theory. In this scenario, dextran-70 produces sufficient physiologic ascites to float mobile tissues and prevent prolonged apposition of healing tissues within the pelvis for more than the three days required for mesothelial regeneration. Crystalloid solutions alone could not accomplish this.

SAFETY ISSUES

Risks associated with the use of high molecular weight dextran-70, marketed in this country as 32% dextran-70 in 10% dextrose, (Hyskon, Pharmacia Inc., Piscataway, N.J.) have generally fallen into three broad categories. Dextran is a derivative of sugar beets, and an allergy to sugar beets and their byproducts could elicit an allergic or even anaphylactic reaction. The vast experience both with intravenous and intraperitoneal use of dextran products as plasma expanders, and as a distending medium in hysteroscopy, tends to suggest that the risk of allergic reaction must be quite small. Although there are scattered reports (Trimbos-Kemper and Veering, 1989), these are anecdotal at best. Ring and Messmer (1977) found the use of intravenous dextran administration was associated with an incidence of only 0.008% anaphylactoid reactions.

In view of the fact that intravenous administration of dextran can prolong coagulation time (Nilsson and Eiken, 1964), dextran treated patients undergoing anticoagulation therapy should be carefully monitored, but the risk in otherwise normal patients appears to be minimal at most.

A significant and realistic concern regards the possible role of dextran-70 in the support of bacterial growth. Once again, the large and relatively benign experience of large numbers of patients who have had potentially contaminated volumes of Hyskon instilled transcervically during hysteroscopy tends to belie this in a practical, clinical sense, but Bernstein et al (1982) did report that Hyskon could support bacterial proliferation. Although it would be reasonable not to consider patients with infected fields as ideal candidates for intraperitoneal dextran therapy, we designed an animal study to test this hypothesis. (Kennedy, Rosenberg, and Gebhart, 1985).In this study LD-50 doses of several common "gynecologic" organisms were injected into mouse peritoneal cavities in the presence of 32% dextran-70, Ringers lactate, and 10% dextrose solutions (the "vehicle" for the dextran in Hyskon). With none of these organisms did the presence of Hyskon, associated with gross peritoneal contamination, increase the previously-determined control LD-50 mortality rates for any of the mouse groups.

SUMMARY

There appears to be significant data both in animal and human studies to support the contention that 32% high molecular weight dextran-70 is of significant benefit in the minimization of surgical adhesion formation--and reformation after lysis. The data would suggest that it is more valuable in more severe cases, and that it tends to be more efficacious in dependent portions of the pelvis supporting, at least in part, the "hydroflotation" theory of its mechanism of action. Allergic reaction is possible but quite rare, and concern about the possible role of dextran-70 in support of clinical bacterial infection appears to be unsubstantiated by both clinical and experimental data.

REFERENCES

1. The Adhesions Study Group: Reduction of postoperative pelvic adhesions with intraperitoneal 32% dextran 70: a prospective, randomized clinical trial, Fertil Steril, Vol.40, No.5, November 1983

2. Bernstein RN, Mattox JH, Ulrich JA, Messer RH: The potential for bacterial growth with dextran. J Reprod Med 27:77, 1982

3. diZerega GS, Hodgen GD: Prevention of postoperative tubal adhesions: comparative study of commonly used agents. Am J Obstet Gynecol 136:173, 1980

4. Holtz G., Baker E., Tsai, E.: Effect of 32% dextran 70 on peritoneal adhesion formation and reformation after lysis, Fertil, Steril 33:660, 1980

5. Hulka JF, Omran K, Berger GS: Classification of adnexal adhesions: a proposal and evaluation of its prognostic value. Fertil Steril 30:661, 1978

6. Kennedy KE, Rosenberg SM, and Gebhart RJ: Effects of dextran-70 on Bacteria-Induced Mortality in Mice. Infertility 8:30, 1985

7. Luengo, J., and van Hall, E.V.: prevention of peritoneal adhesions by the combined use of Spongostan and 32% dextran 70: An experimental study in pigs, Fertil Steril 29:447, 1978

8. Misirlioglu YI, Shafiroff BG: The mechanism of action of dextran-40 and dextran-75 on fibrinogenolysis in vivo and in vitro. The Real Science, May 1973,p 37

9. Neuwirth RS, and Khalaf SM: Effect of 32% dextran 70 on peritoneal adhesion formation Am J Obstet Gynecol 121:420, 1975

10. Nilsson IM, Eiken O: Further studies on the effect of dextran of various molecular weights on the coagulation mechanism. Thromb Haemost (continues Thromb Diath Haem) 1:38, 1964

11. Polishuk WZ, Bercovici B: Intraperitoneal low molecular dextran in tubal surgery. J Obstet Gynecol Br Comonw 78:724, 1971

12. Ring J, Messmer K: Incidence and severity of anaphylactoid reactions to colloid volume substitutes. Lancet 1, 1977

13. Rosenberg SM, and Board JA: High Molecular Dextran in Human Infertility Surgery. Am J Obstet Gynecol Col 148, No. 4 1984

14. Schwartzkopff W: Determination of permeability of the abdominal capillary membranes with low and high-molecular substances. Presented at the Third European Conference on Microcirculation, Jerusalem. Bibl Anat 7:156, 1965

15. Seitz, HM, Schenker, JG, Epstein S, and Garcia CR: Postoperative intraperitoneal adhesions A double-blind assessment of their prevention in the monkey, Fertil, Steril 24: 935, 1973

16. Tangen O, Wik KO, Almqvist IAM, Arfors KE, Hint HC; Effects of dextran on the structure and plasmin-induced lysis of human fibrin. Thromb Res 1:487, 1972

17. Trimbos-Kemper Trudy, Veering B: Anaphylactic shock from intracavitary 32% Dextran-70 during hysteroscopy. Fertil Steril Col 51, No.6, 1989

18. Utian WH, Goldfarb JR, Starks GC: Role of dextran 70 on microtubal surgery, Fertil Steril 31:79, 1979

19. Wallenback IAM, Tangen O: On the lysis of fibrin formed in the presence of dextran and other macromolecules. Thromb Res 6:75 1975

Treatment of Post-Surgical Adhesions, pages 165–175

DEXTRAN - LATER CLINICAL STUDIES

Clinical and experimental evaluation of different adjuvant therapies

Bertil Larsson,M.D.Ph.D.

Department of Obstetrics and Gynecology,
Karolinska Institutet,
Huddinge University Hospital,
Stockholm, Sweden

INTRODUCTION

In 1967 Swolin in Gothenburg published his thesis on microsurgery in tubal reconstructive surgery. In this report a gentle, less traumatic technique was described. This method also included administration of a high dosis of cortisone intaabdominally and for the forthcoming two weeks successively reducing dosis of cortisone, administered per os. This technique is used as routine in Sweden, and so far no complications have been registered. Abroad, however, the administration of cortisone is abandonned and questionned.

So far the mechanism of action in formation of pelvic adhesions is not fully known. It seems, however, clear that previous laparotomies and previous pelvic inflammatory diseases (PIDs) play an important role. According to my own experience, a steadily increasing number of women suffer "silent" PIDs, resulting in infertility due to the tubal factor. Postoperative adhesion seems either to be induced by trauma to the peritoneum, even a slight one, operative or postoperative infection or necrotic tissues. As a certain trauma to the serosa cannot always be avoided, it seems reasonable to use some kind of adjuvant therapy for prevention of postoperative adhesions.

The present review concerns some aspects on the microsurgical technique and adjuvant therapy in prevention of postoperative adhesions.

MATERIAL and METHODS

Sactosalpinges, peritubal- andperiovrian adhesions;

In a series comprising 428 patients, the influence of cortisone, oxyphenbutazone, saline and blood/fibrinogen was evaluated. The distribution of adhesions are summerized in Table 1.

Table 1.

Operations for fertility
N=428

	n	%
Peritubal/periovarian adhesions	36	8
Sactosalpinges	54	13
Sactosalpinges + Peritubal/periovarian adhesions	338	79

Oxyphenbutazone was used in connection with cortisone in 107 patients. The seperate effect of saline and of a slight peritoneal trauma, resulting in areas of petechiae, was investigated in 15 patients of this series and in 15 patients included in the "Hyskon-series".

The amount of blood loss during the operation was

measured by analyse of the towels and registration of the suction amount, and then correlated to the postoperative adhesionscores. The influence of blood and/or fibrinogen was also prior to the clinical study, seperately evaluated inan experimental study in rats (Nisell & Larsson, 1978).

Surgicel - an absorbable hemostatic material - was used in 12 patients. The swabs covered in a singel layer injured serosal areas in pelvis. The series was performed after a study in rats, in which beneficial effects were demonstrated (Larsson et al, 1978).

A two-component fibrin sealant (Tisseel) was used in so far 14 patients in whom tubal anastomisis were performed. In these patients the sealant was used to reinforce the anastomisis and reduce the number of serosal sutures. In 16 patients, serosal defects established after removal of adhesions and due to trauma to the serosa, were covered with a thin layer of Tisseel.

The efficacy of Hyskon (32 % dextran 70) was evaluated in a prospective, randomized, multicenter study including 105 patients (31 patients in Huddinge University Hospital), operated upon for fertility due to the tubal factor (Larsson et al, 1985). At the operation for fertility, including salpingo-neostomy, fimbrioplasty and lysis of adhesions, the type and extent of adhesions as well as the location of the adhesions (oviducts, fimbriae, ovaries, uterus, cul-de-sac, omentum, colon, small bowel, pelvic side wall and abdominal wall) were classified according to a scoring scale (ranging 0 to 4).
The operative procedure was performed throughout the series by the gentle electromicrosurgical technique, previously described by Swolin (Swolin, 1967).
Before closing the peritonel cavity, 250 ml of 32% dextram 70 (Hyskon, Pharmacia AB, Sweden) (n=51), or 250 ml of 0.9 % saline (n=54) was instilled by catheter into the pelvic cavity

according to a random selection system. No other medications, corticosteroids included, were used. All patients received paraenteral antibiotic prophylaxis (tetracycline) during the operation and orally for a week postoperatively. Possible postoperative complications such as infection, bleeding electrolyte imbalance were recorded.
Follow-up laparoscopy with hydropertubation was performed 4 to 10 weeks postoperatively. Intra-abdominal adhesions were recorded and classified according to the same scoring system as used during tubal reconstructive surgery. Tubal patency was also tested.

Tubal anastomosis;

The effect of Salbutamol (a B-adrenergic agonist) was specifically analysed in a series of 17 patients in whom tubal anastomosis were performed. Salbutamol was administered intravenously during operation in one to three dosis of 0.02 mg, until a widening of the tubal lumen was observed with the naked eye. This method facilitated the placement of the sutures in accurate position and intended to advocate the length of the tubal resection until normal tubal tissue was reached.
In tubal anastomisis,cortisone was never used, as it was previously proved to harm the healing procedure.

Follow-up laparoscopy;

The type, amount and extent of the adhesions were registered according to a specific scoring system at the microsurgical operation and compared to the scores registered at the postoperative laparoscopy, performed 2 to 6 months after the operation.

RESULTS and COMMENTS

Experimental studies in rats have demonstrated that cortisone significantly prevents postopera-

tive adhesions (Larsson, unpublished data). In the same series it was also shown that one single high dosis of cortisone, administered in the abdomen, was as effective as long-term treatment with cortisone. When comparing 15 random patients from the cortisone group with the 15 patients included in the saline group in the Hyskon studie, it was evident that treatment with cortisone significantly reduced the postoperative adhesionscores. In our series no complications or side-effects because of the adjuvant therapy with cortisone have been registred.
In order to further evaluate the effect of adjuvant therapy with high dosis of cortisone, we now run a prospective, randomized, multicenter clinical study at 13 different hospitals in Sweden. All included surgeons are fully experienced in microsurgery.

The beneficial effect of keeping the peritoneum constantly irrigated (with saline) for prevention of postoperative adhesions has been demonstrated by us in seperate animal studies (Larsson & Perbeck, 1986).

Evaluating my clinical series it might be clearly stated that blood and/or fibrinogen per se do not induce any formation of adhesions. These observations agree with the results of experimental studies (Nisell & Larsson, 1978). On the contrary, it was concluded that any trauma to the serosa and the presence of necrotic tissues caused adhesions. Moreover, it was observed that trauma to the tubal serosa was followed by heavier adhesions than injures to the serosa of the bowel or the pelvic wall.

Out of the 428 patients included in the microsurgical program, 141 (33 %) got pregnant within a 5-years postoperative time of observation. The outcome of those first pregnancies after operation are summerized in Table 2.

Table 2.
Outcome of the first pregnancy after opertion for fertility in 428 patients.

Pregnant patients	n = 141 (100 %)
-one child	61 (43 %)
-two or more children	25 (17 %)
-spontaneous abortion	36 (26 %)
-ectopic pregnancy	17 (12 %)
-legal abortion	1
sterilisation	1

These results agree with those summerized and published by the author in 1982 (Larsson, 1982).

Surgicel was found to prevent adhesionformation in experimental studies (Larsson et al,1978). However, in clinical evaluations, it was found to be less effective than cortisone, why it was not reasonable to use it anymore.

The use of a two-component fibrin sealant (Tisseel) in operations for fertility, comprising tubal anastomisis and prevention of postoperative adhesions, was evaluated in experimental studies in three species; rabbits, pigs and monkeys, before clinical use. Promising experimental results emphasised further clinical studies. Evaluating 14 patients, it was concluded that the sealant strengthened the tubal anastomosis and thereby reduced the tension on the serosal and muscular sutures, which makes it possible to reduce the number of sutures. When evaluating another 16 patients, it was proved valuable to to cover injured serosa wherby postoperative adhesions were prevented. The fibrin sealant was found not in itself cause adherence after it was set (Larsson et al, 1986).

Intravenous administration of Salbutamol (a B-adrenergic agnoist) during operation was observed to simplify the microsurgical technique of human tubal anastomosis (Larsson, 1984). After administration of 0.02 mg of Salbutamol a 2- to 3-fold increase of the diameter of the tubal lumen was observed with the naked eye. This widening indicated that the tissue was normal, and as verified from histological examinations of resected tissues, without fibrosis or muscular hypertrophy. If the isthmus is not histologically normal, the transport of the fertilized ova might be impaired, and result in infertility. Summerizing the results of operations in patients with muscular hypertrophy and/or fibrosis, support a proposal that those women slowly continue to produce fibrosis in their isthmic parts of the oviduct. Thus, so far none of the patients, not having achieved any pregnancy during the first postoperative year, have experienced any pregnancy during the following two to five years. Moreover, administration of Salbutamol also facilitated the approximation of the lumen and made the operating microscope unnecessary, which is an advantage as an operating microscope is a rather expensive equipment.

The total adhesion score determined at the operation for fertility and at the follow-up laparoscopy in both Hyskon and saline groups were summerized. There was no significant difference in the inital total adhesion score between the two groups. However, follow-up laparoscopy efter the operation for fertility revealed a statistically significant ($p<0.001$) reduction in the extent of the intra-abdominal adhesions in both groups. The adhesion prophylaxis in the Hyskon group, however, was not statistically better han that in the saline group.

The extent of adnexal adhesion was initially similar in both groups and the surgical procedures resultaed in a statistically significant (p<0.00a) reduction of the adhesions. However, there was no difference between Hyskon and Saline groups in this respect.

As regards the extent of adhesion formation in the rest of the pelvis, the initial scores were less pronounced compared with the adnexal adhesions. A decrease in adhesions was observed at the postoperative assessment in both Hyskon and Saline groups and no difference between the two groups could be noted.

Prevention of postoperative adhesions is a major problem in reconstructive tubal surgery. The surgical principles, advocated nowadays, include gentle handling of tissues, meticulous hemostasis an precise tissue approximation (Swolin, 1967; Gomel, 1977) . The avoidance of serosal injury play, accoring to my experience, the most important role in prevention of formation of postoperative adhesions (Nisell & Larsson, 1978).

In experimental studies, dextran instilled intraperitoneally has been demonstrated to reduce adhesion formation (Utian et al, 1979; diZerega et al, 1980). However, results of other experimental studies have not supported these results (Vemer et al, 1982).

In our multicenter study, adjuvant therapy with Hyskon seemed to be without any beneficial effect. Similiar results have been reported in studies where low molecular-weight dextran (Rheomacrodex) solution was instilled intraperitoneally before closing the abdomen (Polishuk & Bercovici, 1971). A significant reduction of postoperative adhesion formation was demonstrated in prospective study where intraperitoneal Hyskon instillation was compared with a control in which Ringer lactate crystalloid solution was used (Rosenberg & Board, 1984). In our multicenter study which was designed in a similar way, no statistically significant difference in postoperative adhesion formation could be observed between Hyskon and saline groups. The different results in these two studies might be due to the fact that in Rosenberg´s study the mean adhesion score was higher in the Hyskon group than in the control group. In a study, designed similar to ours, diZerega et al registered a beneficial effect of Hyskon in prevention of postoperative adhesions (diZerega, 1983).

The reason for the differing results in the experimental and clinical studies are difficult to explain. However, the difference might be due to the different experimental animals, the surgical technique, the localisation of the experimentally induced injury, the dosis of the tested agent and the procedure used in the control group.

One of the most interesting adjuvant agent to be evaluated in ongoing studies is t-PA. Heparin is used at several center of microsurgery, mostly dispersed in the lavage solution.

REFERENCES

Gomel V (1977). Reconstructive surgery of the oviduct. J Reprod Med 18:181-190.

Larsson B (1982). Late result of salpingostomi combined with salpingolysis and ovariolysis by electromicrosurgery in 54 women.
Fertil Steril 37:156-160.

Larsson B (1984). Administration of Salbutamol simplifies the microsurgical technique of human tubal anastomosis. Current Therapeutic Research 35:342-344.

Larsson B, Fianu S, Jonasson A, Rodriguez- Martinez, Hedstrøm KG & Thorgirsson T (1986). The use of Tisseel - a two component fibrin sealant - in operations for fertility as a sealant and for prevention of adhesions. In Schlaug (Ed): "Fibrin Sealant in Operative Medicine", Vienna: Springer Verlag, pp 70-74.

Larsson B, Lalos O, Marsk L, Tronstad S-E, Bygdeman M, Pehrson S & Joelsson I (1985). Effect of intraperitoneal instillation of 32 % dextran 70 on postoperative adhesion formation after tubal surgery.
Acta Gynecol Scand 64:4377-441.

Larsson B, Nisell H & Granberg I (1978). Surgicel - An absorbable hemostatic material - in prevention of peritoneal adhesions in rats.
Acta Chir Scand 144:375-378.

Larsson B & Perbeck L (1986). The possible advantage of keeping the uterine and intestinal serosa irrigated with salin in operations for fertility - An experimental study in rats.
Acta Chir Scand Suppl 530:15-18.

Larsson B, Svanberg SG & Swolin K (1977). Oxyphenbutazone - an adjuvant to be used in prevention of adhesions in operations for fertility 28:807-808.

Nisell H & Larsson B (1978). Role of blood and fibrinogen in development of intraperitoneal adhesions in rats. Fertil Steril 30:470-473.

Polishud WZ & Bercovici B (1971). Intraperitoneal low molecular dextran in tubal surgery.
J Obstet Gynaecol Br Comm 78:724-727.

Rosenberg SM & Board JA (1984). High-molecular weight dextran in human infertility surgery.
Am J Obstet Gynecol 148:380-385.

Swolin K (1967). 50 Ferilitätsoperationen. Teil I. Literatur und Methodik. Acta Obstet Gynecol Scand 46:234-250.

Utian WH, Goldfarb JM & Starks GC (1979). Role of dextran 70 in microtubal surgery. Fertil Steril 31:79-82.

Vemer HM, Boeckx W & Brosens I (1982) Use of dextrans for the prevention of postoperative peritubal adhesions in rabbits. Br J Obstet Gynaecol 89:473-475.

diZerega GS & Hodgen GC (1980). Prevention of postoperative tubal adhesions. Comparative study of commonly used agents. Am J Obstet Gynecol 136:173-178.

diZerega GS et al (1983). Reduction of postoperative pelvic adhesions with intraperitoneal 32 % dextran 70: a prospective, randomized clinical trial. Fertil Steril 40:612-619.

Treatment of Post Surgical Adhesions, pages 177–192

CONTROLLED CLINICAL APPROACHES TO INVESTIGATING THE PREVENTION OF PERITONEAL ADHESIONS

Robert P.S. Jansen

Director of Fertility Services,
Royal Prince Alfred Hospital,
Sydney 2050, Australia.

INTRODUCTION

Adhesion formation competes with mesothelial healing in the delicate equation that shapes the postoperative pelvis. There is no distinction between the two competing processes for the first 3 days after peritoneal injury. A fibrin exudate containing neutrophils and, later, macrophages (Ellis et al., 1965; Raftery, 1973a) first seals the site. Unlike ulcers of the skin or the gastrointestinal tract, which re-epithelialize from their periphery, serosal defects heal from within: new mesothelial cells come mostly from differentiation of the underlying mesenchyme (Clarke, 1915; Ellis et al., 1965; Raftery, 1973b), perhaps partly from seeding by cells of the peritoneal fluid (Bridges and Whitting, 1964; Eskeland, 1966) and only minimally from mitoses at the defect's rim (Clarke, 1915; Eskeland, 1966). A large mesothelial defect therefore heals in the same 7 to 8 days it takes a smaller defect to reperitonealize (Raftery, 1973a; Ellis et al., 1965; Eskeland, 1966).

Fibrin that is not broken down within 3 days by fibrinolysins (present in high concentration in normal peritoneum but often deficient in injured peritoneum) (Myrhe-Jensen et al., 1969; Raftery, 1981) begins to organize, with invasion by fibroblasts and blood vessels (Ellis et al., 1965; Raftery, 1973a; Johnson and Whitting, 1962). Those adhesions that will result are in place by the eight days it takes the mesothelium to regenerate (Johnson and Whitting, 1962; Milligan and Raftery, 1974). By 21 days, adhesions are histologically established, but further fibrosis and contraction continues over many months (DeCherney and Mezer, 1984).

Serosal scarring and adhesion formation is promoted by diathermy coagulation, infection, ischemia, retroperitoneal blood clot, and foreign bodies. Adhesions do not necessarily result from the presence of intraperitoneal blood or from exposing the subserosal mesenchyme (Williams, 1955).

Adhesions generally do not form unless injured and opposing serosal surfaces remain in contact beyond the three-day postoperative point. This is likely (a) if both surfaces have undergone trauma and have become inflamed, (b) if omentum or pelvic fat bodies are in contact with the damaged serosa (it is the omentum's role to attach to damaged peritoneum and to remain attached)(Ryan et al., 1971) or (c) if visceral immobility causes the injured serosa's inflammatory products to poison the previously healthy serosa pressed onto it (Williams, 1955).

The goal of promoting the process of mesothelial healing while suppressing the process of serosal scarring has attracted numerous adjunctive maneuvres, both physical and pharmacological. The goal has proved elusive because these processes are indistinguishable for at least three days after the operation. The literature is replete with such maneuvres that have come into, and out of, fashion. Few have sought to affect peritoneal physiology beyond the three day turning point. Fewer have been subjected to controlled trials in human subjects.

I shall consider these adjunctive maneuvres in relation to several controlled clinical trials monitored by early postoperative laparoscopy and I shall show how the initial extent of the adhesions can unexpectedly bias the outcome of clinical trials if this covariate is not controlled.

VISCERAL MOBILITY

General maneuvres to increase visceral mobility are important and include early postoperative ambulation and an early return to a normal diet (Schiff et al., 1949), Meanwhile the notion has long been attractive that providing a coating or physical barrier between injured serosal surfaces might be useful to avoid or limit the formation of adhesions: the subject was reviewed as early as 1942 (Boys, 1942). Early solutions that met with no success included hypertonic and hypotonic saline, various oils and silicone fluids, air, blood, high molecular weight gelatin and dextrans (Schiff et al., 1949; Ellis, 1971). Natural and synthetic membranes that also met with no success included free omental grafts, amnion, oxidized cellulose and polyvinylpyrrolidone (Ellis, 1971; Connolly and Smith, 1960).

The most popular modern solution to leave in the peritoneal cavity is 32% dextran 70 (Hyskon). Early animal studies on its use were generally encouraging (just about every fashionable solution has been shown to be useful in animals) and a controlled study in monkeys subjected to crush injury of the tubal fimbriae showed Hyskon to be efficacious (DiZerega and Hodgen, 1980). Clinical trials, however, have at best indicated a marginal effect in areas of the pelvis other than the adnexa (Adhesion Study Group, 1983; Rosenberg and Board, 1984; DiZerega and Hodgen, 1980).

To be valid, clinical trials must be controlled for the initial extent of the adhesions. The bias that is introduced by failing adequately to control for this variable is paradoxical. Intuitively one expects that the worse the initial adhesions are, the worse the likely outcome, with or without an adjunct such as dextran (Adhesion Study Group, 1983), but this is not the case. Whatever the system of scoring adhesions one uses, there is a finite limit to the maximum score (the minimum possible score is zero). If the *improvement score* is the final score minus the initial score then the possible range of improvement scores is ± the maximum score.

Plotting improvement scores against initial scores produces a distribution of possible values over an area with the shape of a parallelogram (Figure 1). This plot reveals that the higher the initial adhesion score is, the more likely it is that the improvement score will be positive and not negative; in other words, failing to control for initial scores or, worse, intentionally biasing the treatment group towards severe adhesions may lead to a spurious conclusion that the treatment is efficacious.

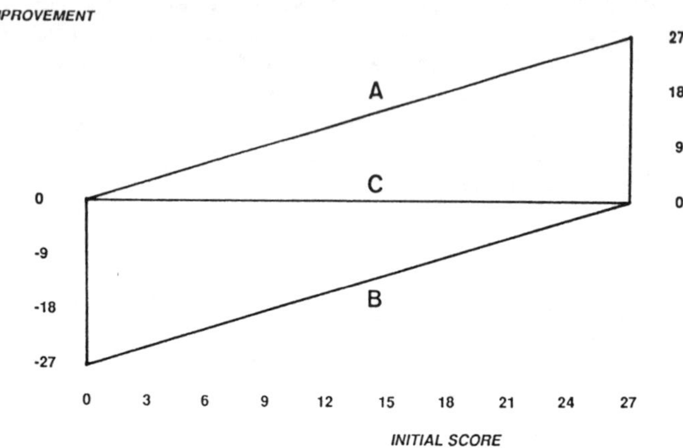

Figure 1. A parallelogram describes the permissible distribution of improvement scores plotted against initial adhesion scores. Irrespective of the system used for scoring adhesions, a high initial adhesion score will bias the outcome in favor of improvement. Line A = best possible outcome; line B = worst possible outcome; line C = no change.

32% Dextran 70

Figure 2 shows the results of a prospective, randomized, controlled, laparoscopically monitored clinical trial of 100 to 200 ml 32% dextran 70 versus a similar volume of Ringer's lactate solution among 164 operations (Jansen, 1985). No benefit is apparent. Clinical stratification and nonparametric comparisons of median adhesion scores at operation and at early postoperative laparoscopy showed in fact that there was a poorer outcome with 32% dextran 70 than when dextran was not used in every subgroup except one (repeat salpingolysis after previous operation for adhesions). A discussion of the other clinical trials involving Hyskon is available elsewhere (Jansen, 1985).

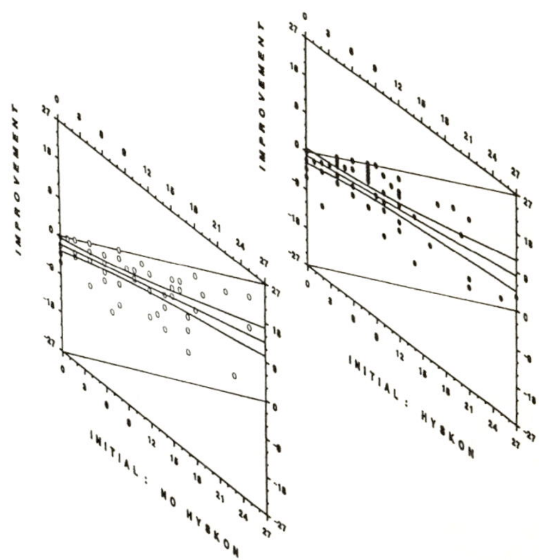

Figure 2. Parallelogram plots of adhesion improvement scores comparing intraperitoneal 32% dextran 70 (Hyskon) against saline controls. Linear regression and 95% confidence limits. The trend is against Hyskon being useful.

The remainder of this paper will use similar parallelogram plots to examine similarly designed clinical trials of other adjunctive measures.

PHARMACOLOGICAL APPROACHES

Pharmacological therapy to promote mesothelial healing over fibrosis and formation of adhesions has a tenuous empirical basis in the clinical practice of preventing adhesions (Connolly and Smith, 1960; Pfeffer, 1980; Jansen, 1985; Jansen, 1988a). Antihistamines (Replogle et al., 1966), corticosteroids (Jansen, 1985; Seitz et al., 1973; Replogle et al., 1966) and antiprostaglandins (Jansen,

1988a) have all been used to tip the balance in favor of healing, but properly controlled clinical studies are few.

Antihistamines

Antihistamines were first used to limit peritoneal adhesions in an experimental study in dogs in 1953 (Berman et al., 1953). Promethazine was used clinically to prevent peritoneal adhesions in 1966 by Replogle et al (Replogle et al., 1966), who administered 25 mg intramuscularly at 6 and 3 hours preoperatively, left 25 mg in the peritoneal cavity at operation, and administered further doses intramuscularly every 4 hours from 2 hours after operation for 24 to 36 hours. In later introducing the regimen to pelvic operations, Horne et al (Horne et al., 1973) administered 25 mg 2 to 3 hours before operation, left 25 mg in the peritoneal cavity at operation, and gave a further 12 doses at 4 hour intervals postoperatively. The duration of therapy in both studies was well short of the 3 days that elapses before fibrosis of unlysed fibrin commences.

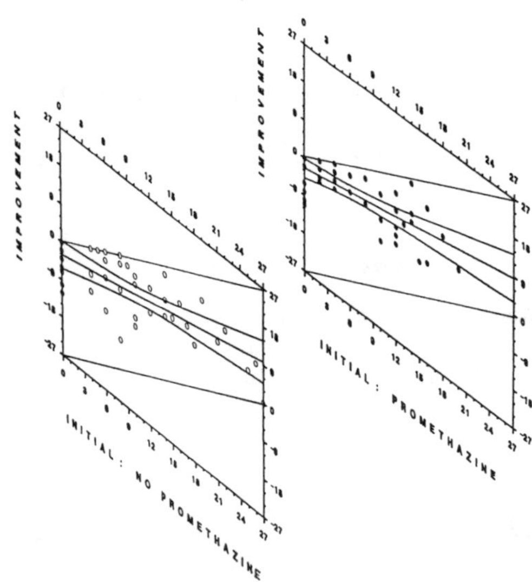

Figure 3. Parallelogram plots of adhesion improvement scores comparing perioperative systemic promethazine against no promethazine. Linear regression and 95% confidence limits. The trend is not in favor of promethazine.

In a recent randomized, controlled and laparoscopically monitored study among 90 patients (Jansen, 1990), 50 mg promethazine was given by mouth 6 to 8 hours before operation) and 50 mg was given intramuscularly during the operation. No beneficial or deleterious effect on the extent of postoperative adhesions was demonstrated (Figure 3).

Corticosteroids

High-dose corticosteroid therapy was used in conjunction with promethazine by Replogle et al (Replogle et al., 1966) and by Horne et al (Horne et al., 1973). In both studies, 20 mg dexamethasone was administered intramuscularly at the same times indicated above for promethazine, and the duration of postoperative therapy was no greater than 48 hours. The combined regimen has been shown to produce short-term suppression of the hypothalamic-pituitary-adrenal axis (Magyar et al., 1984), although the clinical importance of this suppression is doubtful. Complications experienced with the regimen in neonates operated on for bowel obstruction, including wound infection, wound separation and gastrointestinal bleeding (Grosfield et al., 1973), have left infertility surgery in women as the main area in which use of the promethazine-corticosteroid regimen remains prevalent. However, in the only randomized, controlled trial of the combined regimen in primates, Seitz et al found in rhesus monkeys that there was no beneficial effect in preventing the reformation of surgical adhesions (Seitz et al., 1973).

Other studies have employed high-dose corticosteroids intraperitoneally (Swolin, 1967) or systemically (Jansen, 1985) for a week or more after operation, well into the time that fibrosis of unlysed fibrin takes place, with some evidence of efficacy. Controlled trials of slowly-absorbed intraperitoneal corticosteroid formulations are lacking. I have examined the question as to whether the timing of systemic corticosteroid administration in relation to operation and the duration of therapy after operation might be important.

Among 75 patients who received perioperative steroids and a historical control group of 66 patients who did not, there was no substantial difference between adhesion improvement scores (Figure 4) (Jansen, 1990). In these studies dexamethasone 8 to 24 mg was given i.v. during operation and prednisone 25 to 50 mg was given orally before and/or after operation. Other reports indicate that preoperative steroids, to have a significant effect in preventing adhesions, may need to be given for a long time: Cade and Ellis reported that prednisone at a dosage of approximately 1 mg/kg produced a significant decrease in starch-powder induced granulomatous reactions in rats only if started 2 weeks before starch inoculation (Cade and Ellis, 1976).

When systemic steroids in high dosage were confined to the perioperative period, there was no difference between administering steroids 8 hours before operation or 24 hours after operation in a randomized, controlled trial of 75 cases involving mostly patients with low initial adhesion scores (Figure 5) (Jansen, 1990).

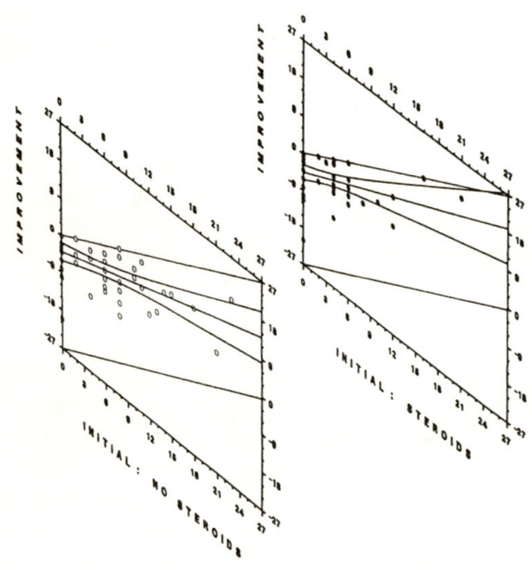

Figure 4. Parallelogram plots of adhesion improvement scores show a trend toward better scores if systemic corticosteroids are administered around the time of operation among patients with high initial scores. Linear regression and 95% confidence limits. The difference is not statistically significant.

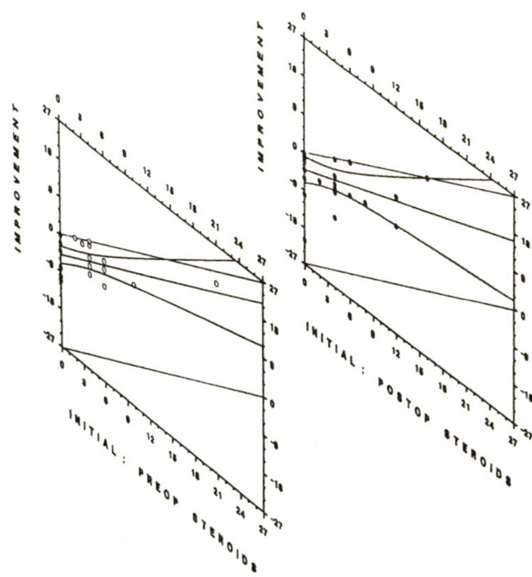

Figure 5. Parallelogram plots of adhesion improvement scores comparing preoperative prednisone versus postoperative prednisone in the same dose. Linear regression and 95% confidence limits. The difference is not statistically significant.

Continuation of systemic steroid therapy beyond the time when fibrosis of unlysed fibrin starts (3 days after operation) until the time of laparoscopy 10 to 12 days after operation was associated with significantly higher improvement scores in a prospective series of 90 cases (Jansen, 1990). Although the difference between the treated group and controls was evident in all subgroups when the study was stratified according to initial adhesion score, the difference was not substantial (Figure 6)

Morbidity associated with prolonged use of steroids was noticeable but slight, with a tendency toward separation of the skin suture line under stress observed in the treatment group.

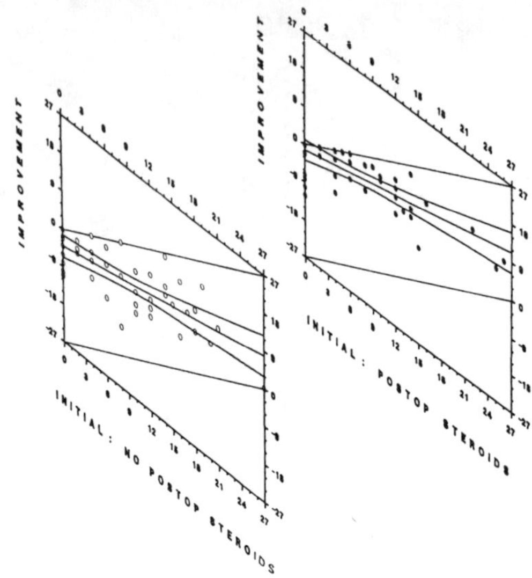

Figure 6. Parallelogram plots of adhesion improvement scores comparing postoperative prednisone therapy for 10-12 days in comparison with no postoperative steroid therapy. Linear regression and 95% confidence limits. Statistically significant differences were demonstrable in subgroups stratified by initial score.

ANTICOAGULANTS

Fibrinous exudation is the necessary precursor to fibrous organization within the peritoneal cavity. Prevention of fibrin deposition and enhancement of fibrinolysis have therefore been attracting attention for many years in attempting to limit development of adhesions. Encouraging reports were published in the 1940s on the use of high dose heparin given intraperitoneally (Lehman and Boys, 1940; Massie, 1945) but complications, including wound disruption and hemorrhage, curtailed its use (Connolly and Smith, 1960; Ellis, 1971). Recently heparin has been used in infertility operations to facilitate accurate microscopic technique unhindered by clotting, as well as hopefully to prevent adhesions. In a further randomized, controlled, laparoscopically monitored trial in 92 patients, intraoperative heparin 5000 units/liter had no beneficial action (Figure 7) (Jansen, 1988a).

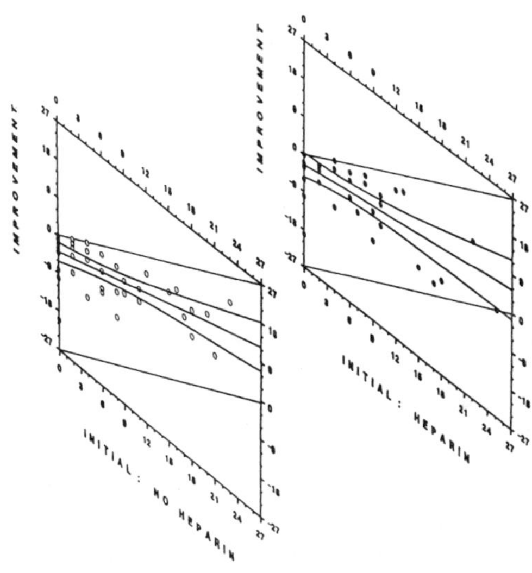

Figure 7. Parallelogram plots of adhesion improvement scores comparing intraoperative, intraperitoneal heparin 5000 u/l with saline controls. Linear regression and 95% confidence limits. The trend is against the use of heparin.

In summary, the only pharmacological adjunct that has yet been shown to work to a statistically significant extent in controlled clinical comparisons has been the use of corticosteroids when administration is extended past the 3-day postoperative point at which mesothelial healing and serosal scarring are distinguishable processes.

More studies are needed on those agents that can be administered beyond the 3-day postoperative point when organization of unlysed fibrin starts. Perhaps the most promising of these is human tissue plasminogen activator (hTPA), available through recombinant DNA technology, and the subject of recent improvements in the treatment of coronary thrombosis. How to put hTPA safely into the peritoneal cavity 3 days or more after laparotomy is a challenge still to be faced.

EARLY POSTOPERATIVE LAPAROSCOPY

Meanwhile, of all available adjunctive drugs and maneuvres, two studies have now shown that a judiciously timed ("second-look") postoperative laparoscopy is an effective way of promoting mesothelial healing over serosal fibrosis and that the extent of pelvic adhesions can, in this way, be significantly and substantially reduced (Trimbos-Kemper et al., 1985; Jansen, 1988b).
The laparoscopy is timed for 8 to 10 days after operation. This is when mesothelial healing is established, but before fibrosis is mature enough to make dissection of the new adhesions difficult. With separation of adherences at 8 days, the proposal is that islands of mesothelium can spread short distances laterally to resurface recently adherent peritoneum before further fibrosis takes place. Morbidity in over one thousand cases has been low (there was one case of infection of intraperitoneal blood and formation of a pelvic abcess), and enough patients have now been evaluated at a subsequent procedure (a "third look") to judge the efficacy of early postoperative laparoscopy.

Figure 8 compares improvement scores achieved in 33 patients from the clinical series referred to above who happened to be examined by a "third look" in comparison with the "second-look" scores of the patients from Figures 2 to 7 (Jansen, 1988b). This comparison shows that early postoperative laparoscopy is presently the most effective available adjunctive procedure to minimize postoperative adhesions.

The efficacy of early postoperative laparoscopy is presumed to follow from its strategic timing, (i) *well* after the 3-day point when inflammation gives way to repair, (ii) *just* after the 8-day point at which mesothelial healing is complete, and (iii) *more or less* before fibrosis is established.

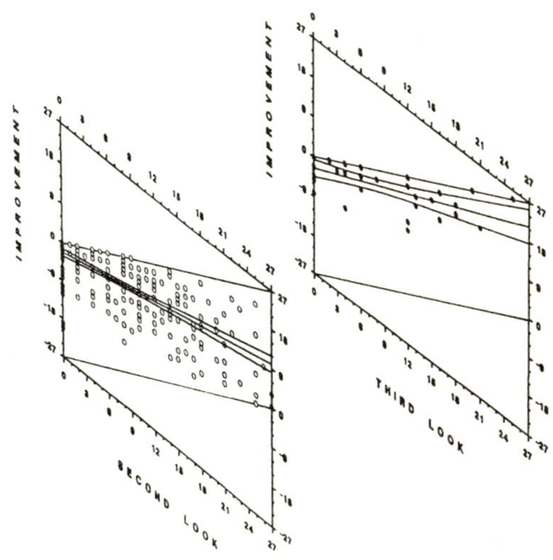

Figure 8. Parallelogram plots of adhesion improvement scores at second-look laparoscopy compared with ultimate improvements obtained by adhesiolysis at second-look as indicated by a "third look". Linear regression and 95% confidence limits. In contrast to the comparisons in Figures 2-7, early postoperative laparoscopy produces a statistically significant and clinically substantial gain in adhesion improvement scores.

It remains to be seen which patients gain most from postoperative laparoscopy, so that its benefits can be weighed against its costs. Meanwhile, the benefits of early postoperative laparoscopy justify its use to monitor future controlled trials of physical and pharmacological measures that extend into the period of dichotomy between mesothelial healing and serosal scarring to minimize pelvic adhesions.

REFERENCES

Adhesion Study Group (1983). Reduction of postoperative pelvic adhesions with intraperitoneal 32% dextran 70: a prospective, randomized clinical trial. Fertil Steril 40:612-619.

Berman JK, Habegger ED, Berman EJ (1953). The effects of antihistamine drugs on fibroplasia. Am Surg 19:1152-1161.

Boys F (1942). Prophylaxis of peritoneal adhesions. Review of literature. Surgery 11:118-168.

Bridges JB, Whitting HW (1964). Parietal peritoneal healing in the rat. J Path Bact 87:123-130.

Cade D, Ellis H (1976). The peritoneal reaction to starch and its modification by prednisone. Eur Surg Res 8:471-479.

Clarke WC (1915). Experimental mesothelium. Anat Rec 10:301-316.

Connolly JE, Smith JW (1960). The prevention and treatment of intestinal adhesions. Surg Gynecol Obstet 110:417-431.

DeCherney AH, Mezer HC (1984). The nature of posttuboplasty adhesions as determined by early and late laparoscopy. Fertil Steril 41:643-646.

DiZerega GS, Hodgen GD (1980). Prevention of postoperative adhesions. Comparative study of commonly used agents. Am J Obstet Gynecol 136:173-178.

Ellis H, Harrison W, Hugh TB (1965). The healing of peritoneum under normal and pathological conditions. Br J Surg 52:471-476.

Ellis H (1971). The cause and prevention of postoperative intraperitoneal adhesions. Surg Gynecol Obstet 133:497-511.

Eskeland G (1966). Regeneration of parietal peritoneum in rats. 1. A light microscopical study. Acta Path Microbiol Scand 68:355-378.

Grosfield JL, Berman IR, Schiller M, Morse TS (1973). Excessive morbidity resulting from the prevention of intestinal adhesions with steroids and antihistamines. J Pediatr Surg 8:221-226.

Horne RW Jr, Clyman M, Debrovner C, Griggs G, Kistner R, Kosasa T, Stevenson CS, Taymor M (1973). The prevention of postoperative adhesions following conservative operative treatment for human infertility. Int J Fertil 18:109-115.

Jansen RPS (1985). Failure of intraperitoneal adjuncts to improve the outcome of pelvic. Am J Obstet Gynecol 153:363-371.

Jansen RPS (1988a). Failure of peritoneal irrigation with heparin during pelvic operations upon young women to reduce adhesions. Surg Gynecol Obstet 166:154-160.

Jansen RPS (1988b). Early laparoscopy after pelvic operations to prevent adhesions: safety and efficacy. Fertil Steril 49:26-31.

Jansen RPS (1990). Effect of perioperative systemic promethazine and corticosteroids on the formation of pelvic peritoneal adhesions. Fertil Steril under review:

Johnson FR, Whitting HW (1962). Repair of parietal peritoneum. Br J Surg 49:653-660.

Lehman E, Boys F (1940). The prevention of peritoneal adhesions with heparin. Ann Surg 111:227-235.

Magyar DM, Hayes MF, Moghissi KS, Subramanian MG (1984). Hypothalamic-pituitary-adrenocortical function after the dexamethasone-promethazine adhesion regimen. Obstet Gynecol 63:182-185.

Massie F (1945). Heparin in the abdomen. Ann Surg 121:508-517.

Milligan DW, Raftery AT (1974). Observations on the pathogenesis of peritoneal adhesions: a light and electron microscopical study. Br J Surg 61:274-280.

Myrhe-Jensen O, Larsen SB, Astrup T (1969). Fibrinolytic activity in serosal and synovial membranes. Arch Path 88:623-630.

Pfeffer WH (1980). Adjuvants in tubal surgery. Fertil Steril 33:245-256.

Raftery AT (1973a). Regeneration of parietal and visceral peritoneum. A light microscopical study. Br J Surg 60:293-299.

Raftery AT (1973b). Regeneration of parietal and visceral peritoneum: an electron microscope study. J Anat 115:375-392.

Raftery AT (1981). Effect of peritoneal trauma on peritoneal fibrinolytic activity and intraperitoneal adhesion formation. An experimental study in the rat. Eur Surg Res 13:397-401.

Replogle RL, Johnson R, Gross RE (1966). Prevention of postoperative intestinal adhesions with combined promethazine and dexamethasone therapy: experimental and clinical studies. Ann Surg 163:580-588.

Rosenberg SM, Board JA (1984). High-molecular weight dextran in human infertility surgery. Am J Obstet Gynecol 148:380-385.

Ryan GB, Grobety J, Majno G (1971). Postoperative peritoneal adhesions. A study of the mechanisms. Am J Path 65:117-148.

Schiff CA, Goldberg SL Necheles H (1949). The prevention of abdominal adhesions. Experimental study on the role of gastrointestinal motility. Surgery 25:257-267.

Seitz HM Jr, Schenker JG, Epstein S, Garcia C-R (1973). Postoperative intraperitoneal adhesions: a double-blind assessment of their prevention in the monkey. Fertil Steril 24:935-940.

Swolin K (1967). Die Einwirkung von grossen, intraperitonealen Dosen glukokortikoid auf die Bildung von postoperativen Adhaesionen. Acta Obstet Gynec Scand 46:1-15.

Trimbos-Kemper TCM, Trimbos JB, Van Hall EV (1985). Adhesion formation after tubal surgery: results of the eighth-day laparoscopy in 188 patients. Fertil Steril 43:395-400.

Williams DC (1955). The peritoneum. A plea for a change in attitude towards this membrane. Br J Surg 42:401-405.

Treatment of Post Surgical Adhesions, pages 193–206

INTERCEED[R] (TC7) AS AN ADJUVANT FOR ADHESION REDUCTION: CLINICAL STUDIES

L. Russell Malinak, M.D.

Dept. of Obstetrics & Gynecology
Baylor College of Medicine
Houston, Texas 77030

Adhesion formation continues to present as a complication in gynecological surgery. The concept of using a physical barrier to prevent adhesion formation has long been attractive. Oxidized regenerated cellulose, a resorbable fabric (SURGICEL[R], Johnson & Johnson Medical Inc., Surgical Specialties Division, New Brunswick, N.J.) was first tested as an adhesion barrier in laboratory animals. In general, those studies demonstrated that Surgicel, as opposed to many foreign bodies, did not promote adhesions when left in the abdominal cavity after surgery [Galan (1983), Hixson (1986), Larsson (1978), Nishimura (1983), Raftery (1980), Schroder (1982), Shimanuki (1987), Soules (1982), Yemini (1984)]. The physical properties of Surgicel were then redesigned through prototype development and preclinical testing to provide a material that could cover traumatized tissues and act as a barrier to the formation of adhesions; INTERCEED[R] (TC7) Absorbable Adhesion Barrier was the result. Interceed (Johnson & Johnson Medical Inc., Surgical Specialties Division, New Brunswick, N.J.) is a fabric composed of oxidized regenerated cellulose specifically designed as a surgical adjuvant to reduce the formation of post surgical adhesions. Additional preclinical studies with Interceed demonstrated that (1) it promoted negligible tissue response, (2) this new material completely absorbed from the peritoneal cavity in less than 28 days, (3) it reduced the extent and severity of post surgical adhesions in standardized animal models, and (4) was compatible with laparoscopic application in large animal surgery [Diamond (1987) (1989), Linsky (1987)].

We report the clinical evaluation of Interceed in the first 74 patients of a multi-center study as an adjuvant for adhesion formation in patients undergoing gynecological surgery [Interceed Study Group (1989)]. In addition, preliminary results on the final study group of 134 patients will also be described.

Principal investigators and study site were: Ricardo Azziz, M.D., University of Alabama at Birmingham, Birmingham, Alabama; Stephen Cohen, M.D., University of Massachusetts Medical Center, Worcester, Massachusetts; David N. Curole, M.D., Fertility Institute of New Orleans, New Orleans, Louisiana; Michael P. Diamond, M.D., Yale University School of Medicine, New Haven, Connecticut; Robert R. Franklin, M.D., Texas Woman's Hospital, Houston, Texas; Arthur F. Haney, M.D., Duke University Medical Center, Durham, North Carolina; L. Russell Malinak, M.D., Baylor University College of Medicine, Houston, Texas; Wayne S. Maxson, M.D., Northwestern Medical Plaza, Margate, Florida; Grant W. Patton, M.D., Southeastern Fertility Center, Charleston, South Carolina; John A. Rock, M.D., The Johns Hopkins Hospital, Baltimore, Maryland; Sanford Rosenberg, M.D., Richmond Center of Fertility, Richmond, Virginia; Bobby W. Webster, M.D., Center of Reproductive Medicine, Wichita, Kansas; and A. Albert Yuzpe, M.D., University Hospital, London, Ontario, Canada.

From July 1986 to August 1989, infertility patients in 13 investigational centers underwent elective laparotomy for lysis of bilateral pelvic sidewall adhesions. All study sites had Institutional Review Board approval and patients gave informed consent.

Excluded were patients under 18 years of age, those with cancer, those without a tube or ovary, and those who had irrigants/instillants containing 32% Dextran 70 (Hyskon, Pharmacia, Piscataway, N.J.), corticosteroids, non-steroidal anti-inflammatory agents. Also excluded were patients with hematological or coagulation disorders. Adhesions were evaluated throughout the peritoneal cavity with specific attention focused on both lateral pelvic sidewalls. When attached to sidewalls and organs, the adhesions were described and graded as I (filmy), II (organized, vascular), and III (cohesive).

The data was recorded on standardized forms for computerized data reduction. Drawings and photographs were taken to document operative findings.

Various modes of adhesiolysis were carried out. These included sharp dissection, electrocautery, or laser, with or without magnification. The extent of deperitonealized surface was described and its area measured. Operations performed in addition to lysis of adhesions were resection, fulguration of endometriosis, salpingostomy, tubal anastomosis, and myomectomy.

After completion of all operative procedures and establishment of complete hemostasis by microelectrocautery, laser or suture, a sealed envelope disclosed assignment of treated and untreated sidewalls. Interceed was applied in an amount sufficient to completely cover all deperitonealized surfaces on the sidewall indicated by the randomization plan. The contralateral sidewall was left uncovered, thereby serving as the control.

The assignment of test sidewall (either left or right) for each patient was performed prior to the beginning of the study by the sponsor who used a computerized algorithm to insure randomness. A separate randomization was generated for each investigational center. Patient numbers were randomized in blocks of two to provide balance with respect to left and right sidewalls. The algorithm was supplied by Digital Equipment Corporation, Maynard, Massachusetts, as a Fortran system subroutine.

Interceed was supplied as a sterile unit of 7.6 cm x 10.2 cm. After cutting to the appropriate size Interceed was placed on the deperitonealized surface and readily adhered to the tissue without suturing. Where appropriate, the material was wetted with a small amount (about 1 ml) of irrigation fluid to provide additional tack.

Patient demographics, etiology of adhesions, and methods of hemostasis are presented in Table 1.

TABLE 1

STUDY POPULATION AND DEMOGRAPHICS

	MEAN	RANGE
AGE (Yrs.)	29	(19-38)
RACE	NO.	%
Caucasian	62	84%
Black	10	13%
Hispanic	2	3%
PRESUMPTIVE DIAGNOSIS ADHESION ETIOLOGY		
Unknown	37	50%
Infection	23	31%
Endometriosis	7	9.5%
Prior Abdominal Pelvic Surgery	7	9.5%
REPRODUCTIVE HISTORY		
Gravida		
0	38	51%
1	27	37%
2	9	12%
DIAGNOSIS		
Pelvic Adhesive Disease	48	65%
Tubal Occlusion	17	23%
Endometriosis	7	9%
Pelvic Inflammatory Disease	2	3%

A second-look laparoscopy for evaluation of pelvic adhesions was performed between 10 days and 14 weeks after the laparotomy. Findings and data recording were carried out in a manner similar to that at laparotomy.

Three characteristics of adhesions were used to assess efficacy: (1) incidence of adhesions, defined as the presence or absence of adhesions at "second-look" laparoscopy; (2) extent of adhesions, which required measurement of the deperitonealized area on the pelvic sidewall postadhesiolysis at the time of laparotomy and the same area at laparoscopy; (3) severity of adhesions which subjectively evaluated the tenacity or strength of the fibrotic bands as well as the presence of vascularity within the adhesions. Severe adhesions (Grades II and III) were organized bands which did not provide planes for surgical dissection and were frequently vascular. Filmy adhesions were transparent and easily removed.

Two parameters were utilized to evaluate the extent of adhesions: (1) area measurements of deperitonealized tissue on the pelvic sidewalls at the time of laparotomy and laparoscopy, as well as (2) organ involvement and adhesion resolution. Reduction was expressed as: (a) area reduction i.e. the pretreatment area (laparotomy) minus post-treatment area (laparoscopy); (b) percent improvement was the above area reduction divided by pretreatment area x 100; (c) differential percent improvement = percent improvement due to Interceed minus the percent improvement due to microsurgery alone.

The feasibility of combining the data between study centers was assessed by employing a one-way analysis of variance. Because patients were utilized as their own control (Interceed covered versus noncovered sidewalls), the paired t-test was selected as appropriate for paired dependent observations. The non-parametric counterpart of the paired t-test was employed to evaluate results that may give concern relative to their underlying parametric assumptions. Relationships between baseline variables and effectiveness measures and the uniformity of baseline variables among study centers were examined in two-way contingency tables employing chi-square tests. McNemar's Test was used to evaluate the results of the "absent/present" response since patients served as their own control. Levels of significance correspond to a two-sided alternate hypothesis. A p value less than 0.05 was chosen to indicate statistical significance.

Application of Interceed was randomized to the right sidewall in 39 (53%) of the patients and to the left sidewall in the other 35 patients. An analysis of variance (p=0.8) showed the consistency and feasibility of combining data over centers. Since all patients were enrolled under the same protocols and there were no clinical observations that contradicted pooling of the data among investigational centers, the results were combined for matched-pairs analysis.

Significantly more adhesions were observed (Table 2) at second-look laparoscopy on the control side, 53 of 74 (72%) cases, than on the treated side, 34 of 74 (46%) cases (Chi-Square, p=0.003). Fourteen patients had no adhesions on either sidewall (Column III); 27 patients had adhesions on both the control and the Interceed treated sidewalls (Column IV). In 26 patients, adhesions were present on the control sidewalls when there were no adhesion on the Interceed treated sidewalls (Column I). In seven patients, adhesions were present on the Interceed treated sidewalls when there were no adhesions on the control sidewalls. When post-treatment adhesions were absent on one sidewall and present on the contralateral side, Interceed had a significantly greater number of cases without adhesions (26 versus 7 cases). This difference in matched-sidewall comparisons is highly significant (p=0.0003, McNemar Test). Interceed treatment eliminated the formation of adhesions in nearly twice as many pelvic sidewalls as adhesiolysis alone (40 versus 21) representing a 90% improvement over microsurgery alone in preventing adhesions.

TABLE 2

MATCHED-PAIR COMPARISON OF THE ABSENCE OR PRESENCE OF SIDEWALL ADHESIONS AT LAPAROSCOPY

	I	II	III	IV
Interceed(TC7)	-	+	-	+
Control Sidewall	+	-	-	+
First 74 patients	26	7	14	27
134 patients	46	10	22	56

+ = Adhesions Present
- = Adhesions Absent

When the preliminary analysis for the final group of 134 patients was performed, the above conclusions were further substantiated with the larger population. Interceed prevented adhesions in over twice as many patients [68 (46+22)] as did the control [32 (10+22)]. Furthermore, utilizing a matched pair comparison for only those patients showing a difference in treatment outcome (Columns I and II), the treatment outcome was 4.6 times greater than that of the control (46 vs 10).

The mean deperitonealized area for all the sidewalls (n=148) at laparotomy and at laparoscopy is demonstrated in Table 3. The area of the control sidewalls involved with adhesions decreased from 8.8 cm^2 (range 0.3 to 54 cm^2) to 3.1 cm^2 (range 0 to 12 cm^2); the size of the Interceed treated sidewalls decreased from 10.8 cm^2 (range 0.25 to 70 cm^2) to 1.6 cm^2 (range 0 to 15 cm^2). Sidewalls treated with Interceed had significantly less area involved with adhesions compared to surgery alone (p=0.004, paired t-test).

TABLE 3

SIDEWALL AREA (MEAN)

	LAPAROTOMY	LAPAROSCOPY	DIFFERENCE
Interceed	10.8	1.6	9.2
Control	8.8	3.1	5.7

The reduction in the amount of sidewall area that was reduced by the procedure performed at laparotomy. The mean area reduction for Interceed treated sidewalls was 9.2 cm^2, whereas the mean area reduction for the control sidewalls was 5.7 cm^2. It is noteworthy that though the Interceed group had a larger denuded surface area than control sides at laparotomy, the adhesions were smaller in the treatment sidewall than the control sidewall at the time of second-look laparoscopy.

In order to adjust for variation in pretreatment areas of the Interceed and control groups, the percent improvement scores were evaluated. The area difference was normalized with respect to the initial area, then multiplied x 100. The overall percent improvement in sidewall areas involved with adhesions was 82% for Interceed and 58% for the control. These differences are highly significant (p=0.001, paired t-test). When all 134 patients were analyzed, this difference was further substantiated (76% vs 56%, $p < 0.0001$).

The differential percent improvement was determined to assess the effectiveness of Interceed in reducing the extent of adhesions relative to surgery alone. This method adjusts to eliminate possible bias due to differences among patients at laparotomy. It first takes the percent improvement per sidewall adjusted by the initial area. Next, it matches the difference between the sidewall percent improvements for each patient (i.e. matched-pair). Whereas the percent improvement evaluates the overall change, the differential percent improvement goes one step further and matches the sidewalls. The overall mean differential percent improvement was 24%, which is highly statistically significant (p=0.0001, determined by both the paired t-test and Wilcoxon Signed Ranks test). Thus, Interceed provided a 57% improvement in reducing the extent of adhesions over that provided by surgery alone. This improvement was calculated as the ratio of the improvement seen (24%) over the amount of improvement possible in excess of the control.

The number of adhesions was similar for both groups at laparotomy, though there were fewer adhesions on Interceed sidewalls at laparoscopy. Both treatment and control groups had comparable distribution of organs involved in adhesions. Only the ovaries had sufficient numbers of adhesions for statistical analysis. The results of matched-pair analyses show that 25 patients had sidewall-ovarian adhesions on the control side, at laparoscopy (Column I), with no sidewall-ovarian adhesions on the Interceed treated sidewalls (Table 4). In contrast, there were only five cases where sidewall-ovarian adhesions were absent on the control sidewalls, and present on the Interceed treated sidewalls. Reduction in the number of cases with sidewall-ovarian adhesions by the application of Interceed was significantly different from that achieved by surgery alone (Table 4, p=0.0003, McNemar Test).

TABLE 4

ABSENCE OR PRESENCE OF SIDEWALL-OVARIAN ADHESIONS AT LAPAROSCOPY

	I	II	III	IV
Interceed Sidewall:	-	+	-	+
Control Sidewall:	+	-	-	+
Ovary after treatment	25	5	19	25

+ = Adhesions Present
- = Adhesions Absent

Severity of adhesions was the third parameter of efficacy evaluated. Severity was subjectively determined by assessing the tenacity or strength of the fibrous bands and the vascularity of the adhesions. Adhesions emanating from the sidewall to various organs were quantified before adhesiolysis. Thus, on a given sidewall, one to several filmy and/or severe adhesions could be recorded. Table 5 shows the total number of filmy adhesions noted at laparotomy for the Interceed and control groups. Of the 31 filmy adhesions at laparotomy, 27 did not reform at laparoscopy, three remained filmy, and one was severe. The majority of these filmy adhesions did not reform in both the Interceed treated (87%) and control (68%) groups. Table 6 shows that there were over twice as many adhesions at laparotomy in the severe category as compared to the filmy type (85 versus 31). A significant benefit was seen for Interceed over surgery alone in reducing the number of "severe" adhesions (Chi-Square, p=0.028).

TABLE 5

FILMY ADHESIONS - OUTCOME AT LAPAROSCOPY

	INTERCEED	CONTROL
Laparotomy	31	34
Laparoscopy		
None	27 (87%)	23 (68%)
Filmy	3 (10%)	8 (23%)
Severe	1 (3%)	3 (9%)

TABLE 6

SEVERE ADHESIONS - OUTCOME AT LAPAROSCOPY

	INTERCEED	CONTROL
Laparotomy	85	77
Laparoscopy		
None	56 (66%)	35 (45%)
Filmy	15 (18%)	19 (25%)
Severe	14 (16%)	23 (30%)

The correlation between time to second-look laparoscopy and outcome was also evaluated. The data do not support a correlation between adhesion formation and the interval between laparotomy and laparoscopy performed 10 days to 14 weeks after adhesiolysis (r=0.003). The assessment of outcome was therefore not affected by the interpatient variation in the time interval between laparotomy and laparoscopic evaluations.

Studies on synthetic absorbable barriers to reduce adhesion formation are limited; except for oxidized regenerated cellulose (Surgicel), the methods reported resulted in more adhesions than untreated controls. Larsson (1978) first suggested that a knitted fabric made of this material might be a promising agent in the prevention of cecal adhesions. Raftery (1980) found it prevented peritoneal adhesion formation in rats. Galan

(1983) reported its beneficial effect in reducing adhesions using a rabbit uterine horn reanastomosis model. Finally, it was shown to provide a graded reduction in adhesion formation after uterine trauma and intestinal anastomosis [Nishimura (1983), Shimanuki (1987)] in standardized animal models.

However, not all studies demonstrated efficacy in prevention of adhesions. Schroder (1982) evaluated Surgicel among other modalities and failed to demonstrate efficacy in preventing cecal adhesions in rats. Yemini (1984) also reported no benefit by the use of Surgicel to prevent adhesion reformation in a rat uterine horn model. Soules (1982) found that Surgicel application offered no advantage over no treatment after a standardized cut or scrape of the rabbit uterine horn. Hixson (1986) studied the ability of Surgicel to prevent postsurgical adhesions to the fimbria and ovaries; here, also, Surgicel showed no activity for preventing adnexal adhesions.

The mixed results of these reports indicate that Surgicel is noninflammatory, supports re-epithelialization after tissue injury, and is bioabsorbable; nonetheless, the above studies showed that its properties as an adhesion barrier needed redesign. Accordingly, a wide variety of fabrics composed of oxidized regenerated cellulose in animal models of adhesion formation were tested. The knit, weave and porosity which maximally prevented adhesion formation were identified and combined to formulate the product Interceed.

When compared to untreated controls, Interceed significantly reduced postoperative adhesion formation to the lateral abdominal sidewall of rabbits compared to untreated controls [Diamond (1987)]. Interceed placed on the deperitonealized surfaces of both the sidewall and uterine horn of rabbits significantly reduced adhesion formation [Diamond (1987), Linsky (1987)]. No complications from the use of Interceed were reported in these studies. The fabric was absorbed from the peritoneal cavity at two weeks.

Larsson (1978) suggested that oxidized regenerated cellulose affects the process of adhesion formation by its transformation into a gelatinous mass that covers the damaged peritoneum and thereby protects it from involvement in adhesion formation. Interceed rapidly forms a soft gelatinous mass which provides a protective coating around healing tissue during the initial seven to 10 days after application [Diamond (1987), Linsky (1987)]. During this time, re-epithelialization of damaged peritoneal surfaces is completed.

In these preclinical studies, the presence of blood significantly reduced the efficacy of adhesion barriers such as Interceed [Linsky (1988)].

To obtain maximum benefit, it is essential to achieve complete hemostasis prior to applying the material. Application of the barrier was most efficacious after irrigation of the peritoneal cavity just prior to closure to reduce the possibility of Interceed displacement.

This clinical study was designed to assess the safety of Interceed intraperitoneally and its efficacy in prevention of adhesions which occur secondary to pelvic surgery. The primary inclusion criterion was the existence of adhesions on both pelvic sidewalls. This allowed each patient to serve as her own control, enabling matched-pair comparisons. Laparoscopy was performed 10 days to 14 weeks after adhesiolysis to evaluate three determinants of efficacy: (1) incidence, (2) extent, and (3) severity of the adhesions identified at the initial laparotomy.

Good surgical techniques (control) prevented adhesions in 28% of the cases. In contrast, Interceed, when combined with good surgical techniques, resulted in adhesion prevention in 54% of the cases (Table 2). Hence, Interceed was nearly twice as effective in preventing adhesions when compared to surgery alone. Moreover, in a matched-sidewall comparison, Interceed was nearly four times (35% versus 9%, Table 2) more effective in preventing adhesions when compared to the contralateral sidewall (surgery alone).

The adhesions were analyzed by area differentials, percent improvement scores, and differential percent improvement scores. While all three approaches lead to the same conclusion, the differential percent improvement score is the most precise because it adjusts to eliminate possible bias due to differences among patients at laparotomy. The percent improvement evaluated the overall changes, whereas the differential percent improvement went one step further and matched the sidewalls. The combined differential percent improvement for Interceed over the control sidewall areas was 24%, which was statistically significant. In addition, Interceed provided a 57% improvement in reduction of the overall extent of adhesions. Sixty-one percent of adhesive attachments were pelvic sidewalls to ovaries. Interceed was shown by matched-pairs analysis to significantly prevent the formation of ovarian adhesions to the pelvic sidewall after surgery. Also, it significantly reduced the severity of the adhesions formed. Thus, Interceed offered additional improvement over microsurgical techniques alone in reducing the incidence, extent, and severity of postoperative adhesions. Additionally, preliminary analysis of 134 patients further strengthened the conclusion of the first 74 patients.

In conclusion, Interceed Adhesion Barrier effectively reduced the incidence, extent, and severity of postoperative adhesion. INTERCEED, in conjunction with meticulous hemostasis and gentle tissue handling, provided a useful adjuvant to state-of-the-art surgical techniques. With its recent availability to the gynecologic profession, the role of INTERCEED as an adjuvant in the reduction of adhesions will become further defined.

REFERENCES

Diamond MP, Cunningham T, Linsky CB, DeCherney AH (1989). Laparoscopic application of Interceed(TC7) in the pig. J Gyn Surg 5:145.

Diamond MP, Linsky CB, Cunningham TJ, Constantine B, DeCherney AH, diZerega GS (1987). A model for sidewall adhesions in the rabbit; reduction by an absorbable barrier. Microsurgery 8:197.

Galan N, Leader A, Malkinson T, Taylor P (1983). Adhesion prophylaxis in rabbits with Surgicel and two absorbable microsurgical sutures. J Reprod Med 28:662.

Hixson C, Swanson LA, Friedman CI (1986). Oxidized cellulose for preventing adnexal adhesions. J Reprod Med 28:662.

Interceed(TC7) Adhesion Barrier Study Group (1989) -- Prevention of post-surgical adhesion by Interceed(TC7) an absorbable adhesion barrier. A prospective randomized multicenter clinical study. Fertil Steril 51:933.

Larsson B, Nisell H, Grandberg I (1978). Surgicel -- an absorbable hemostatic material -- in prevention of peritoneal adhesion in rats. Acta Chir Scand 144:375.

Linsky CB, Diamond MP, Cunningham TJ, Constantine B, diZerega GS, DeCherney AH (1987). Adhesion reduction in the uterine horn model using an absorbable barrier, TC7. J Reprod Med 32:17.

Linsky CB, Diamond MP, DeCherney AH, diZerega GS, Cunningham T (1988). Effect of blood on the efficacy of barrier adhesion reduction in the rabbit uterine horn model. Infertility 11:273.

Nishimura K, Bieniarz A, Nakamura R, diZerega GS (1983). Evaluation of oxidized regenerated cellulose for prevention of postoperative intraperitoneal adhesions. Jpn J Surg 13:159.

Raftery A (1980). Absorbable hemostatic materials and intraperitoneal adhesion formation. Br J Surg 67:57.

Schroder M, Willumsen H, Hart Hansen JO (1982). Peritoneal adhesion formation after the use of oxidized cellulose (Surgicel) and gelatin sponge in rats. Acta Chir Scand 148:595.

Shimanuki T, Nishimura K, Montz FJ, diZerega GS (1987). Localized prevention of postsurgical adhesion formation and reformation with oxidized regenerated cellulose. J Biomed Mater Res 21:173.

Soules M, Dennis L, Bosarge A, Moore P (1982). The prevention of postoperative pelvic adhesions: An animal study comparing barrier methods with dextran 70. Am J Obstet and Gynecol 143:829.

Index